Boyfriend University

Boyfriend University

Take Advantage of Your Man and Learn While You Can

JENNIFER SANDER
and
LYNNE ROMINGER

WILEY

John Wiley & Sons, Inc.

Published by John Wiley & Sons, Inc., Hoboken, New Jersey
Published simultaneously in Canada

For general information about our other products and services, please contact our Customer Care Department within the United States at (800) 762–2974, outside the United States at (317) 572–3993 or fax (317) 572–4002.

Wiley also publishes its books in a variety of electronic formats. Some content that appears in print may not be available in electronic books. For more infor-mation about Wiley products, visit our web site at www.wiley.com.

Library of Congress Cataloging-in-Publication Data:
Sander, Jennifer.
  Boyfriend university : take advantage of your man and learn while
you can / Jennifer Sander and Lynne Rominger.
    p. cm.
  Includes index.
  ISBN 978-0-470-17703-7 (pbk.)
  1. Women—Life skills guides. 2. Achievement motivation in women.
  3. Women—Psychology. I. Sander, Jennifer Basye, date. II. Title.
  HQ1221R714 2009
  646.70082—dc22   2008041536

Printed in the United States of America

10 9 8 7 6 5 4 3 2 1

To all the men I've learned from,
my heartfelt thanks.
—Jennifer

For my baristas, Jeremy,
Keyan, Meghan and Jessica.
Thanks for the shots!
—Lynne

Contents

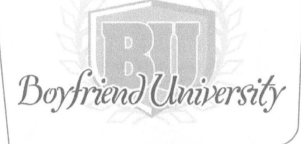

GETTING IN AND CAMPUS LIFE

Do you remember your first date? Your first big love affair? The machinations of men and women can be difficult to navigate sometimes. Just starting the process of getting into a relationship is as daunting as the application process for getting into a university. Once you start a new relationship, it's like starting a new school. Relax. In part I, we give you all the info you need to get into the scene and feel comfortable.

1

An Introduction to Boyfriend University

Jennifer's young son Julian loves to tell his friends, "My mama was a race car driver." As you might imagine, this gets mixed reactions from the other moms: raised eyebrows, knowing looks, amused nods. It's clear that they all believe she has an imaginative child. So sweet that he thinks of his mama that way, though . . .

Jennifer will tell you that Julian is an imaginative child indeed, but he didn't make it up. You might not guess from watching her help out in a grade school class, but yes, she was a fully licensed race car driver. Ladies, start your engines! Jennifer's top speed as a driver was just a hair above 150 mph. As a passenger, she's been in cars going as fast as 180.

Why did she learn how to race? Take quick turns without crashing? Feel the thrill of a powerful, roaring engine? Simple: she had a boyfriend who raced cars.

Lynne is a tall, dark-haired gal who loves both fine literature and fine handbags. Not only can she expertly apply kohl eyeliner and false eyelashes, she can also shoot a weapon like an army sniper and call an NBA game like a referee. Yep, Glock and AK-47 skill and free-throw know-how were both acquired because of boyfriends.

We both attended what we like to call "Boyfriend University" (BU for short). Readers, we see you nodding. You went to that school, too, didn't you, and you know *exactly* what we're talking about. We're guessing there is a thing or two you know how to do because of someone you dated, right?

From the time we're little girls, we're told, "If you want a boy to like you, take an interest in his hobbies. Ask him about himself. Learn to like what he likes." Sound familiar?

Over the years we got a lot of guys to talk about themselves. Jennifer took an interest in their hobbies; she learned to like what they liked. Lynne had a more devious approach. She secretly found out her boyfriends' interests and then threw herself into gaining the skills to impress them and their families.

Jennifer didn't get married until she was thirty-five, so she went to this school for twenty long years, and her course list is *long*:

Racing 101

I learned to operate high-performance vehicles on professional tracks. This was fun! I confess, I love to drive fast, and I learned how to do it safely. Give me pencil and paper and I'll draw the turns on any of the West Coast racecourses like Laguna Seca and tell you how to drive the fastest line around those curves. It is a science of sorts, one of the many things Lynne and I share with you in *Boyfriend University*. But I liked the driving suit best. Have you seen how sexy those race car drivers look in them? Mine was tailored, light blue with white stripes up the side. And the cool thing? My helmet was black—nothing pink for me. On the back it said "A+." No, that's not the grade I got in driving school; it's my blood type. That way if I was pulled unconscious out of a flaming wreck the emergency crew would have that information. By the way, knowing how to control a car at high speeds still comes in handy these days: my husband likes me to drive on long road trips so they don't take as long.

Middle East History
I had many professors on this topic. Ask me anything about the Saudi royal family, prerevolutionary Iran, or even the once-vanished-but-now-returned country of Armenia. One ex-beau recently attained a very impressive-sounding diplomatic post. He is now Armenia's ambassador plenipotentiary to Europe ("envoy" in plain English).

Introduction to English Antiques
Thanks to a date or two with the impressively named Gaylord, I know quite a bit about how to assess the value of English furniture from the sixteenth and seventeenth centuries. I quickly discovered that the fastest way to learn about the value of an item was to measure the strained sound of his voice as I reached out to touch something.

After a stint at Boyfriend University, Lynne was married briefly in her midtwenties, then went right back to school. Some of her courses include:

Advanced Military and Law-Enforcement Weaponry
Do you know the difference between mortar and flak? A rifle and a gun? Here's a little rhyme from my Marine boyfriend, Staff Sergeant Tyler Keagy*, whom I dated upon his return from Operation Desert Storm. It will help you remember that there is indeed a difference between what a soldier fights with and what a cop carries in his holster: "This is my weapon. This is my gun. One is for shooting. The other's for fun!" Shooting master

---

*Some of the names in this book have been changed.

Keagy showed me how to fire safely and effectively and how to identify different weapons. I'm proud to say that when I later encountered a creepy guy who threatened me, I was able to confidently say that he'd better stay away from my home or I'd pull out my Glock. It's one thing to say *gun*, it's another thing to know the name of a specific and powerful make of a handgun. Needless to say, the creepy guy stayed away.

Introduction to Slavic Culture and Cuisine

Ah yes, Radko Pavlovic! His name alone was reason enough to date him, but what I learned about Serbian history enabled me to speak confidently on air about the Serbo-Croatian and Serbo-Kosovar conflicts in the late 1990s—a decade after our dating days. Moreover, to impress his family when we were together, I joined a Serbian dance group and learned to "Kolo" like crazy. (Kolo is the traditional Serbian national folk dance.) I danced so well that I traveled with the troupe and performed all over California. I also leaned to cook traditional Serbian cuisine, like torte (a layered dense and sweet cake) and *gbinica* (a cheese pie).

Contracts 1A/Contracts 1B

What my former boyfriend Walter Warden may have lacked in humor, he made up for in teaching me the important aspects of contracts. Especially the importance of inserting the word *reasonably* everywhere possible in order to always ensure a way to negotiate what the term means. And reading the fine print. I took notes when he reviewed contracts for me and even balked when he wanted a contract between us for a joint project we did (but I now see, after a deal gone bad, just how right he was). Always get a contract if possible. I should mention that I got interested in military intelligence and history because he was an intelligence officer before going to law school.

Naturally there were a number of sports courses that we both took—baseball, tennis, scuba diving, rock climbing. Do you need to know how to fill out those little squares on a baseball scorecard? Jennifer sat in the bleachers watching a blond boy named Greg play all throughout seventh and eighth grades, so she can show you how. What does that batting average number really mean? Lynne can answer that—she dated a major-league baseball player. Scuba diving? Jennifer has logged many hours of underwater time, most of it spent trailing after one fellow whose idea of the buddy system in diving was "same day, same ocean."

And then there are the odd little things we each picked up while attending BU: how to flip two tortillas at once; government regulations for sealed floors in a food manufacturing plant; how geckos mate. Call us if those questions ever come up in a game of Trivial Pursuit, and we'll be happy to fill you in.

Do we sound a tad too manly with all these interests? Trust us, we're both as girlie as they come. Yes, we laud the idea of learning what we can from men. We want women to absorb the useful information available to them but never to abandon their own genuine interests and hobbies. Our ultimate goal in gathering as much information as possible from the men we dated was to *grow*—to grow ever more successful, more smart, more self-assured. We have never expected our relationships to complete us, only to enhance our lives.

For centuries, smart and sexy women have existed and thrived—women who haven't been afraid to use to their advantage the very things that make them different from men. And they have reached their goals and accomplished their dreams everywhere from the boardroom to the bedroom. We're not advocating that you all become Mata Haris. Far from it! What we espouse takes intelligence and the nurturing of one's femininity. It is both a feminist and a feminine approach to life. You take everything you ever learned from a man and use it to your advantage. From shooting a weapon to downing tequila shooters—use it! You become more learned and intelligent with each relationship. You become more adept and skilled and more confident and savvy about the world around you with each boyfriend. Smart and sexy women know that to achieve everything they've ever desired, they must study the characteristics of what they desire. What do you say? Are you with us?

2

How to Use This Book and Why You Should

So where do you go with all this knowledge? How can attending Boyfriend University help you in life and in love?

We authors like to call ourselves "fuzzy-sweater feminists": women who are both beautiful *and* strong. And trust us, we aren't advocating that you subjugate yourself at all! Never. But we do advocate using your God-given abilities to your advantage. After all, don't men use their masculinity—their leverage—in business all the time? They use their ability to "fight the battle" and win. They use their strengths— whether it's the power of their muscles or the power of their words—to achieve what they want. Why shouldn't we women use our power and strengths as well? Why shouldn't we use what men can teach us to further our skills and talents, too? We can. We did. Now it's your turn.

Much of what we've learned from men has been invaluable. When Jennifer feels shy, for example, she simply mimics former flame Cub Trujillo, sticks out her hand to a stranger, and boldly says hello. When she feels wary, she remembers her old beau George and quietly observes and gathers information. Concerned that she might get caught doing something she ought not to be doing, she pretends to be her former friend Scott and smiles blithely while apologizing for not understanding the rules.

Jennifer's habit of learning from men has helped her become more self-reliant. Some might cringe at the throwback idea that women need to learn from men. Both of us think it has exposed us to far more useful things than we ever learned hanging out at the mall with girlfriends. We both adore our women friends, but they didn't show either of us how to stand up on a surfboard, change a tire, or use a kitchen knife properly. That's not to imply that we women don't share and help one another learn every day! Our female friends provide us with different perspectives and lessons. But as women, we're sort of the same "bird." Some of the things we learn from one another come more naturally than what a man can teach. That's why we wrote this book. *Boyfriend University* is about all the useful things and the handy knowledge that men can teach us.

In order to graduate from Boyfriend University, you must absolutely reject the notion that to be smart, capable, and independent a woman must also be unattractive and undesirable, an unfortunate stereotype that we hope to obliterate. This book is for women who want to cultivate both their intelligence and their beauty—and take all the good from every relationship they enter! Most important, don't change for a man—change for yourself instead.

Here's where the fuzzy-sweater-feminist thing comes back into play. In a way, we're on a mission with *Boyfriend University* to help women see the difference between displaying their bodies for attention and using their gender, the characteristics intrinsic to their DNA, to their advantage in the business world and in the bedroom. BU graduates are smart and sexy women who love their bodies and brains while breaking through the glass ceiling and enjoying men!

We've added four types of sidebars with unique and interesting information—making the courses even more fun to attend. These sidebars are particularly important because we realize that sometimes you might be between boyfriends and still want to take an elective or two at BU. For those trying times, we've devised these "slacker courses" within many of the lessons.

Caution keeps you from getting taken and helps you stay safe. In some incidences, you might need to maneuver a little differently than outlined in the chapter or need some extra cautionary advice on a topic.

Extra Credit displays added information on the topic being covered. EC is knowledge that only the best students learn!

Put Your Knowledge to Work provides tips on how the information you have just learned can help you succeed in your career.

Film Studies showcases great moments in cinema where a female character learns something from a man and uses it later to her advantage. Remember, for example, the scene in *Titanic* where Rose finally learns to spit properly? It sure came in handy later on! We've got lots of great examples that require nothing more than popping in a DVD, sitting back on the couch, and enjoying the show.

We didn't set out to write a relationship book, but we've been in relationships, so we'll give advice to readers through some of these lessons, particularly in the discipline of "Biology and Chemistry," with sections titled How to Accept Pleasure and When to Sleep with a Guy. Each discipline provides added tidbits that give readers ways to improve their relationships. Having difficulty understanding your man? You might visit "Communications Studies" first. See, not only does this book provide you with practical lessons on everything from how to kick in a door to how to jumpstart a car, but it also offers classes that'll help your relationships with men flourish. Why? Because you'll be better armed to react, act, and speak with men on their level; you'll get insight into how they were nurtured psychologically compared to how we were. Yep, so much of anything in relationships comes down to nature vs. nurture. Men and women are different animals (nature) and we're treated differently and taught to respond differently as children (nurture). We'll clarify enough about this topic to help you everywhere from work to pleasure (and, yes, we mean physical, sexual enjoyment).

We'll show you how to be a "taker" in a positive way, and teach you how *not* to get used in relationships, how to feel daring and successful without a man, and how to move from man to man in these times of casual dating without any bitterness at the end of the road. Speak up and ask the man in your life: "Teach me!" "Show me!" Then let him show you, and if need be, walk away proudly and do it yourself . . . then impress your next date with your incredible knowledge of pro basketball, fly-fishing, or the Great War. Why not adopt our slogan: I came. I dated. I conquered.

So how are these Boyfriend University skills organized? To help you decide what classes you'd like to take, we've grouped the lessons into three parts that contain facets of campus life and broad areas of discipline (or areas of study). Right now you're reading part I, "Getting In and Campus Life," which covers your freshmen orientation (or introduction) to Boyfriend University. It includes the chapters "Financial Aid and Administrative Offices" (which includes How to Shrug Off a Loss and How to Deal with Men and Loans), "Counseling Services" (with the classes How to Feel Daring and Successful without a Man and How to Know If He's a Fixer-Upper and Worth Keeping, among others), and "Leaving

Home and Living on Your Own" (which includes How to Control a Skid, How to Properly Pound a Nail, and How to Carve a Turkey).

Part II, "Finding Your Major," is divided into the chapters "Art and Cultural Studies" (with the sections How to Bluff and Flatter, How to Drink Cognac, How to Get a Tattoo You Won't Regret, and so on), "Communications Studies" (with lessons in subjects like How to be a Team Player, How and When to Call Men, and How to Feign Interest in a Much Younger Date), and finally, "Biology and Chemistry" (with courses like How to Pick Up a Guy, How to Hide Bad Behavior, and more).

Part III, "Extracurriculars," includes the chapters "Studying Abroad" (with lessons such as How to Find the North Star and How to Breeze through Security) and "Spring Break and Summer Vacation" (which includes How to Play Beer Pong, How to Plan the Perfect Weekend, and How to Play Poker).

In the same way that relationships are random, so is the information in BU. Who knows what you might learn today? Some information you might need right now in your life; other info might turn out to be necessary in the future. But you will soon learn to chop an onion without crying, use the NATO phonetic code, or accept pleasure without guilt, all in one afternoon. Because life and love are like that, aren't they? You just never know what the next moment (or the next man, for that matter) will bring. . . .

3

Financial Aid and Administrative Offices

So much of what we learned from our "businessy" boyfriends came in handy later on. Things like negotiation, compromise, and being authoritative. Sometimes we turned right around and used those skills on them, in order to negotiate our way out of an argument or authoritatively state our desires. Nothing wrong with using business skills in your love life, girls.

Business skills also come in handy when dealing with money. We all know women who seem to fund their men endlessly, but does that mean that you should, too? Money is a touchy topic in relationships, and you need to be able to deal with it skillfully. Acquiring stuff together can also get sticky if the relationship unravels. Our section on How to Deal with Mergers and Acquisitions will help you handle that.

After reading the skills in this section, you will be able, if necessary, to shake your ex's hand firmly and walk away, shrugging off the loss and looking forward to a new beginning.

How to Have a Firm Handshake

All of Jennifer's businessmen boyfriends were first-class handshakers; not a limp grip among them. Every time she turned around they were sticking out a hand and introducing themselves, or greeting a friend, or making a new acquaintance. Putting your hand out to a stranger or a friend seemed like such a natural gesture as a result, but it took her awhile to master the skill. Given her druthers she'd much rather give a half smile and a short nod to acknowledge someone else. But we live in a world of handshaking, so we'd all better get used to it.

What's with all this handshaking anyway? Spend any time at a Renaissance fair (or with a guy who belongs to the Society for Creative Anachronism) and you will soon learn that much of today's etiquette comes from the days of yore when most men carried weapons. Shaking hands upon meeting someone is an ancient way of showing someone that you are unarmed and bear him no harm. Why the right hand? Because if you have your right hand out it means you can't be holding your sword in it. Or a dagger, for that matter.

Boyfriend University Firm Handshake Rules

1. Look the person in the eye and extend your right hand without hesitation (hesitation spoils the effect).

2. Continue looking directly at that person, not at anyone else, and don't break your gaze until the shake is done.

3. Clasp your other hand over the person's hand for a more feminine touch. Jennifer uses this when she's acknowledging that the other person has done her a favor but she doesn't want to say it out loud.

4. Shake at least two times, but not more than three unless the other party keeps going.

When your meeting is over, or the social occasion has ended, if you started out with a handshake you will need to offer it again as you part. No, you don't have to go around the room hunting down everyone whose hand you've been shaking, but put it out there to whomever you are having your last conversation with as you are headed out the door. Look the person in the eye again and say sincerely, "Good to meet you!"

PUT YOUR KNOWLEDGE TO WORK

Always place a name tag on the right-hand side of your shirt in a social setting. This is an old political trick that Jennifer learned in her early career as a lobbyist. If everyone puts his or her name tag on the right, it's easier to see the tag as both people put out their right hands to shake, and they can pretend that they know each other's name. "John! Good to see you again!" It is a great help to those of us with faulty memories.

How to Shrug Off a Loss

Does this sound familiar? You learn that an ex-boyfriend is seemingly unfazed by the fact that you dumped him. Or he's untroubled by the fact that he dumped you. How can men be so blasé about it, dusting themselves off and moving on, while we women sit around for months and years still sniffling over the one who left us behind? Or how about a work setback that you are still smarting over weeks later? Or the fact that someone else managed to get her hands on the last pair of jeans in your size just as you were reaching for them? What guy would be brooding over any of this?

Jennifer has realized that some of this ability comes from sports. Just like the team-building skills some of us didn't pick up, the ability to move on after things haven't gone our way is another lesson we might have learned on a sports field had we spent more time there. Win, lose, win, lose—the fact is, if you lose enough times, you get used to it.

Jennifer finally mastered the ability to let go of defeat and look forward to the next contest (of any kind) after spending time on the racetrack. How could anyone work so hard, build up such anticipation, lose big-time, and then walk away untroubled?

Who likes to lose? No one, really. Not men, not women; even small children are annoyed when things don't turn out as anticipated. But we are all better served by the ability to shrug off losses, both big and small. And if you weren't born with the innate ability to move on, here is some advice Jennifer gleaned at the track: We can't control everything, so the outcome is never really in our control. That is the hardest thing to accept sometimes, particularly for women. We think that if we just try hard enough to make things perfect—particularly when it comes to relationships—that everything will turn out just fine. And then when it doesn't, we blame ourselves and brood over what we did wrong, how we should have done it differently, how if we just had a second chance to try again . . . We play those tapes over and over again in our heads, which further keeps us from moving on after a loss or a defeat.

You need to simply acknowledge that you did the best you could, it didn't go your way, and now you need to leave it behind you so that you can get ready for life's next challenge. As Jennifer's race car boyfriend once said immediately after a stunning loss, "I don't have time to get upset. I have to start getting the car ready for next week's race." Yes, this lesson is short, but so is the message: get over whatever (or whomever) it is and move on.

How to Make Conservative Investments

Every woman should know how to make her money grow. The money rules Jennifer was schooled in from financial men in her life were easy: Make it. Keep it. Grow it. The making it part was okay; the keeping it part could be hard when she was more interested in spending than in saving. But then once she did indeed save, how to make that money grow? Slowly and conservatively, was the advice she got. The world is full of dazzling-sounding ways to make fast money, but don't even try.

What every woman needs are dividends. Stocks that pay out a share of the company profits to their shareholders every year can help your portfolio grow steadily.

With so many choices when it comes to buying stocks, how do you decide which one to trust will increase in value over time? Here are a few important ingredients for solid stock selection:

Understand the product or service the company provides. Sit in a Starbucks and you know that they sell coffee. Use an HP printer and you understand at least one of the products they make. Don't get swept up in some hot-sounding stock from a company that does something you can't quite put your finger on.

Do your homework. Investigate the management of the company by reading the annual report and news releases, as well as analysts' opinions to ensure continuity in performance of the stock price.

Choose only companies whose stock you can see owning for the long haul. Trendy stocks can crash and burn, whereas solid companies can produce year after year.

Be smart in choosing the price you are willing to pay for quality. Cheap stock? Maybe there is a reason it's so cheap. Expensive stock? Maybe there is a reason for that, too.

When working with professionals, be sure that they answer your questions and are courteous—don't give your money to rude people. As with any other relationship, leave quickly if your needs aren't being met.

A few other smart and simple money moves you should be practicing are to always, always, always put the maximum into your company 401(k), particularly if they match. Why pass up free money? And why squander money you already have? As more than one frugal man pointed out to Jennifer, it is better to rein in your spending and hang on to what you already have rather than have to earn the same money over again to just keep up with the bills.

How to Negotiate a Discount on Anything

Just as we sometimes have trouble getting to the point, we women also don't always have the fortitude to get in there and try to strike a better deal. Jennifer watched her boyfriend Cub Trujillo bargain for amazing things, even hotel rooms. She learned that whether it is a house, a car, a raise, or a pair of amazing blue jeans, it never hurts to ask.

The meek may inherit the earth, but the bold will buy it back from them at a reduced price. Want to save money day in and day out on the things you buy anyway? Then speak up and ask for a better price. Even small reductions in price can add up to large yearly savings and let you hang on to more of your money. Rest assured, when you speak up and ask for a better price, you aren't being rude; you're being savvy. Here are four ways to broach the subject anywhere, anytime:

1. I've been a loyal customer for years; are you offering any special deals for new customers that I should know about?

    It does seem more than a bit ironic that a new customer would get a better deal than someone who has been using the product or service for years. It happens all the time, though, in the world of magazine and newspaper subscriptions, health clubs, cable companies, and cell phone plans. So whenever you see a new deal offered from a company you already work with, call up and ask if they can offer it to you, too. Make some noise about how unhappy you are to be penalized for your loyalty, suggest that you might take your business elsewhere or cancel the service, and don't be surprised if you end up with something to make you feel better. Go ahead and ask this question of anyone you've been loyal to over the years: your dentist, your auto mechanic, or your children's piano teacher.

2. Is this the best you can do on the price?

    A perfect way to ease into getting a better deal, this simple question is a polite, but not pushy, way to ask for a discount. It works best in a bazaar-type setting like an antiques and collectibles fair or a big outdoor craft event; anyplace where you are dealing face-to-face with a decision maker. Ask the question, smile expectantly, and then wait. Resist the urge to talk until the other person has spoken. Successful negotiation requires silence.

3. Does this item go on sale anytime soon?

    Few things in life are as annoying as making a big and important purchase only to learn that the very same thing went on sale for half price the next day. So always ask about planned sales before you pay full price for anything. Some stores will go ahead and make the sale right away with the reduced sale price; others will let you put your items on hold until the sale

21

begins. If a store won't do either, you can always put the item back and take your chances that it will still be there when the sale begins.

4. Do you have any of these in the back that have been returned? Many major retailers like Sears and Best Buy routinely take returns from their customers and then are willing to sell the returned items to someone else at a discount. Perhaps the display box was damaged, or there is a tiny scratch. Ask about "open box" items, which are returned merchandise that is slightly used. You can also ask to buy the floor model at a reduced price. This works in electronic stores and office-supply stores with televisions, laptops, and appliances. Furniture stores will also sell floor models for less than the full retail price.

If you begin to add these four questions to your daily life, you will soon see a difference in how much you pay for things. The bottom line is this: you won't get a better deal unless you ask for one. The worst thing that can happen is being told no. The best

PUT YOUR KNOWLEDGE TO WORK

Okay, so you make an offer—"Would you take $800?" The most important thing to know is the need to be quiet. Stop now and wait for the other person to talk. You've just made an offer; hush up and let him or her make the next move. All too often (and Jennifer has succumbed to this frequently) the tendency is to get nervous when there is silence and start talking again before the other person does. And when you do talk, you will undercut your own deal. "Well, actually, I could go up to $875; would you take that?" Whereas if they countered at $900, you could have gone down to $875. Now you are stuck going upward from there, aren't you?

thing that can happen is to save a part of what you were going to spend anyway. Don't be meek; be bold and ask away!

Many stores will refund you the difference between the regular price you paid for an item and the sale price they just advertised a few days after you bought yours. March back in there and hold out your receipt and tell them they need to bring a smile to an unhappy customer's face.

How to Reach a Compromise

Compromise? What's that? Giving something up in order to reach an agreement? Not what any of us really wants to do now, is it? But we have learned (over and over again) in both life and love that sometimes it is the only way to move forward. No amusing boyfriend anecdotes to share here, mainly because we don't want you to know just how often we compromised over the years! But should you need to compromise somewhere in your life sometime, too, here are a few things we picked up along the way.

Sometimes, feelings and emotions are just too high for a compromise to be reached. What to do then? Leave it alone, Lynne has learned. Let everyone cool off and then try again.

There are many reasons to compromise in life—to settle a disagreement, to come to terms in a business situation, or to get some sleep. And when attempting to compromise, you need to decide just how much you are willing to give up in order to come to an agreement.

So you will need to go in with the following two things:

1. An idea of what you want

2. An idea of what you might be willing to give up to get what you want

When approaching a business situation, it isn't a bad idea to ask for more than what you really want in order to be able to settle on the number you actually hope you can get. And hey, maybe you will get more anyway!

Should you ask for more in a personal situation, in the hopes of getting what you actually want? Should you say you want to do dinner and a movie on Friday night, hoping that you will get to go to the movies? Well, we think you are better off saying what you want in those situations, rather than resorting to games.

"We're just going to do it my way," says deal maker George Bingham more often than not. You have to be in a strong position to say that, though, he cautions. If you truly believe that you have the stronger position, go ahead and stand firm for what you want. Understand that there are people out there, both in business and in life, who won't be willing to reach a compromise with you. "Sometimes I outline two parts of a deal and tell the other party to go ahead and choose one. There are two halves of the business apple; which one do you want? You choose one, I'll take the other. And sometimes, they still ask for more than their half of the apple!" George continues. How to deal with these folks? Either be willing to live with a deal you think is unfair, or be willing to walk away. It is up to you.

CAUTION
Should you compromise? Women tend to do it a lot. So maybe every so often you should decide you aren't going to compromise—you won't take anything less than your stated selling price on your great-aunt's dresser, you don't want to see any movie other than the one you've chosen, and no way is cubic zirconium at all close to a real diamond.

And if it doesn't go your way, hey, we already taught you how to shrug off a loss, so you can handle it.

No one reads minds. Not your boss, not your boyfriend. So if there is something you want, speak up and ask for it. You won't get what you don't ask for. Scary as it is to open your mouth and put it out there, you need to speak up. And once you have stated what you want, let the negotiations begin!

How to Stay Organized

Lynne's friend Liz has the world's neatest younger brother, Stew. An investment specialist, Stew is unusually organized. He seems to attract organized friends, too. Both of his male roommates, a firefighter and a tile contractor, are almost as organized as he is. Lynne and Liz visited these twentysomethings and found an immaculately clean and organized house—even the kitchen! They peered in every cupboard, giggling in astonishment at how organized and packed they were. Every dish, pan, and plate, the silverware, and even the food had a logical spot and was put away neatly. Nothing sat in the sink. There was even a cupboard for tea and coffee! All three men parade women in and out of the house. It's no wonder—they're babe magnets!

How do Stewie and his friends stay so organized and clean? Liz says that that even as a toddler, Stew habitually straightened out the throw rugs and the remote controls on the end table in the family room. Lynne's found that many successful men she's dated (and one she married) tend to be organized. Jennifer notes that all those nice men who could pack cars so well also kept tidy offices! Check out this section to see how these men stayed organized and how you can apply their tips to keep yourself from getting buried under clutter.

Who doesn't want to find a way to streamline his or her life and stay organized? The world is in constant chaos and moving toward more chaos (we're talking physics here, folks). It's up to us

PUT YOUR KNOWLEDGE TO WORK

In chapter 6, "Art and Cultural Studies," we teach you how to fake a clean house. You can read ahead and put your knowledge to work if you want to appear organized when the boss pays an unexpected visit to your messy office. Use our tips in How to Fake Your Way to a Clean House and fake a clean office instead!

to continually keep things in order. Some people find this an easy endeavor. Others, not so much. In the business world, staying organized can make the difference between getting the bid and losing the bid. Not to mention, who wants to pick up after someone all the time? What follows are many ideas given by highly successful men as to how you, too, can stay organized:

- Even if you think you are disorganized, never refer to yourself or describe yourself to others as "disorganized" or "messy." If you say it, you will become it. Instead, say that you're the most organized person around!

- Commit to getting organized; it doesn't just happen.

- Keep your appointments on a calendar, whether it's on your computer, your BlackBerry, your cell phone, or in a good, old-fashioned day planner. Stewie couldn't possibly keep up with all his clients and meetings without listing them on a calendar.

- Do what needs to be done right away. For example, if the faucet breaks, get on it! Go to the hardware store, pick up the supplies you need, and immediately get to work. Stew's former brother-in-law taught him the old adage "Never put off tomorrow what you can do today," which leads us to our next tip.

- Ignore the section How to Procrastinate in chapter 6. Procrastination typically is in opposition of organization. Sure, there are times you'll want to procrastinate, but generally, in your business dealings especially, don't.

- "Go through your mail every day," says Stew. Whereas Lynne's dad will let his mail pile up day after day, if you walk into Stew's house, you won't see any envelopes or junk mail around. After he reads an advertisement, he throws it away.

- Put a system of organization in place that works for you. The neat freaks at Stew's house don't walk on the carpet in their shoes (dirt, ya know!), so they've designated a place in the entryway for all footwear. Lynne's had a hook by her door ever since dating a guy who did the same. Why? Because she puts her keys on the hook each day when she comes home and never loses them that way.

- Put things back in their place, no matter what. If you take a book from a shelf, put it back on the shelf. If you cook with a pan, clean it and put it away. (This is a pet peeve of Stew's; you'll never find a pan on his stove if it isn't in use.)

- Throw away, donate, or recycle something most every day. No matter how small, something's got to go! Not only will you clear your house of clutter and help yourself stay organized, but you'll also receive a tax deduction for your donations.

- Consider a less materialistic approach. How much stuff do you really need?

- Ever seen those guys with the hyperorganized tool areas in the garage? All the drawers of the toolboxes neatly filled, all the tools hung cleanly on the wall? Lynne's ex-husband, Tyler, kept his tools in neat side-by-side boxes. Lynne realized that she could organize her large shoe collection the same way Tyler did, in long, plastic crates, which she then slid under the bed. Now her shoes are immaculately organized by color and style.

How to Deal with Mergers and Acquisitions

Mergers and acquisitions? No, we can't really teach you how to acquire a company. We mean merging your things with someone else's things, and perhaps acquiring other things together. This topic belongs in the Boyfriend University School of Business because you need to approach it in a businesslike manner. Because when you try to undo some of those mergers and acquisitions at the end of a relationship, well . . . it doesn't always go so smoothly. Jennifer learned the hard way when an ex hung on to her old British sports car for two long years after she'd moved on. He wouldn't let her take it out of his garage because he decided that she owed him for work he'd done on the car. The lesson? Always make sure that things are spelled out and carefully understood. You might not always need to get it in writing, but at least have the conversation.

> **CAUTION**
> When a man's feelings are hurt—like Jennifer's car-mechanic boyfriend—he may sometimes try to hurt you back. He may become difficult and insist on keeping something he knows you want. You'd be stunned at how often pets are in the middle of breakup struggles. In order to settle things, you might just have to recognize the emotion and move on without your object in order to end the struggle. Jennifer did finally get her car, but only after her ex's feelings had healed and he was ready to move on, too.

Over the course of a relationship you will no doubt buy something together or combine your own things in some way. It's lovely to buy an old painting together at an antiques shop during a romantic weekend getaway or drag your extra sofa over to his house because he really needs one. And as long as you are together, it will continue to be lovely. But there might come a time when things aren't so very lovely and you want your sofa back and you like the way that painting looks in your living room, not his. How to settle these things? Start by looking at these two criteria:

1. **Who paid?** If one person paid for something, even if you chose the painting together at that little antiques store, then, emotion aside, that person is the rightful owner. If you both pitched in and paid together, you own a percentage and should offer to buy the other person out. Much like a co-owned business in which there is a buy-sell agreement in place for the partners to use when they break up, one person has the right to buy the other one out.

Lynne's lawyer boyfriend taught her to insert the word *reasonably* wherever you can in any kind of agreement, so it will be open to interpretation. Not a bad thing to know.

2. **Was it a gift?** Gifts are yours and don't have to be returned. But if it ends up as a huge hassle, you might be better off returning it anyway in order to end the fight. Remember to focus on what you want, which is to end the relationship. The longer a disagreement over stuff goes on, the longer it will take for you to get this guy out of your life for good.

How to Deal with Men and Loans

Some men like to give money (or so we hear), and some men like to borrow it. What to do when your boyfriend taps you for cash? Will you ever see it again?

Three men—Lynne's father, her great-uncle, and her former husband—significantly affected the way she views lending money to friends. They each held a slightly different perspective—as in what circumstances in which to lend—but maintained similar perspectives regarding how a loan might impact the friendship. Interestingly, her father's influence led her to send cash through the mail to a starving Marine fifteen years ago. Just out of college in her first job, Lynne took her last $60 and sent it to the man she'd soon marry. She'd only known him for a short time, so why did she do it? Because her father lived by the credo that when someone is in need, you give—and you don't expect it back. Let's look now into whether that's good advice and also at some ways to ensure that your friendships and relationships don't end over finances.

Money issues are one of the leading causes of any breakup. Follow these tips learned from a few wise guys regarding friendship and lending money:

- As mentioned above, Lynne's dad always gave if asked. And he also never expected to be reimbursed. "In my mind I consider it a gift," he says. "That way, if it is returned, I'm surprised and elated. If it's not, I never harbor hard feelings toward my friend."

    To act in this manner, however, requires that you look closely at whether you can *comfortably* afford to lend the sum

PUT YOUR KNOWLEDGE TO WORK

Did you know that if you give a personal loan to a friend for more than $10,000 you are required to charge interest? Check with your tax person regarding the specific laws and paperwork if you find yourself in this situation.

being asked. When Lynne loaned her fiancé her last few dollars for the month, she had gas, food, and shelter. It didn't cause her a hardship. However, a few years earlier, she actually gave the money for her car payment to a friend to buy a new dress for a Christmas party, thinking that she'd get the money back. She didn't, and she had to scramble to meet her monthly obligations. She decided that day to follow her dad's example. She wouldn't deny anyone—but only if it didn't impact her own finances negatively. Before you lend any money, ask yourself, "Can I do this comfortably? What will the impact be on my finances if I don't get reimbursed?"

- Lynne's great-uncle also lends money but expects to receive it back. In fact, he tells anyone taking money from him, "It'll be here for you again in a time of need if you pay it back." He lets friends know that if they pay him back, he'll always help them out. But if they default on the loan, they'll never see a penny from him again. You might want to consider Lynne's uncle's perspective, which can keep freeloaders from returning.

- When Lynne's ex-husband lends money, he always puts the details in writing, including the repayment plan. That leaves no question about the money being returned. On the downside, when he's not paid, the friendship ends. This man will take his friends to small claims court if necessary. Interestingly, an ex-girlfriend of his borrowed $5,000, never paid it back, and then declared bankruptcy on the debt. Just a forewarning about lending money: you might lose a tidy sum and never get it back.

Simply put, the best thing to do regarding money is to decide whether you comfortably can loan the funds and what the terms of the loan are. You have to be able to live with that decision, whether it's thinking you'll never see the money again or losing the friendship in court. Perhaps the best advice of all again comes from Lynne's dad: never ask for a loan from a friend or a relative unless you write him or her a postdated check that you know will be good the day it's cashed. She never has.

How to Act with Authority

Although Jennifer's boyfriend Cub Trujillo was younger than her, in many situations she often felt as though she was the younger one, because he presented himself to the world with such amazing confidence and authority. While still in his early twenties, he ordered around a crew of men much older than himself in his contracting business—"Here's what I need you to do, here's when I need you to do it, here's how I want you to do it." Jennifer was in awe of his ability. How did he learn that so early in life? "I just act as if I know what I'm doing," he said, "and it seems to work every time."

Say you are suddenly in a leadership position and you don't feel too leaderlike. What to do? Act as if you know what you are doing. That is the advice many inspirational speakers give about achieving success: just act as if you already are successful and pretty soon you will be. Not a bad way to act with authority. Act as if you

> **CAUTION**
>
> When acting with authority, never, ever end a sentence with the question "Okay?" This implies that you are asking a question rather than stating what you want. If you are giving a directive, or an order, or some sort of strong suggestion, ending with "okay?" implies that your wishes are open to discussion. Imagine this: in the heat of battle a general says, "We are going to go in there and roust the enemy no matter how hard it is, no matter how long they fight, no matter what it costs us, okay?" Kind of dilutes the strength, doesn't it?

have authority, act as if you expect people to follow your lead, and many times they will. Here are some tips:

1. Sound like you know what you are doing.

Women tend to not have authoritative voices. Perhaps it's too high or too thin, or perhaps we succumb to that tendency to drift off toward the end of our sentences and not actually finish what we . . . meant to say. Or worse, we end our sentences in a higher pitch than when we started so that there is a singsong quality that undercuts the seriousness of our points. So focus on keeping your voice even and not letting it drift into the higher registers toward the end of what you are saying. Stand in front of the mirror and practice this; it might take some getting used to. And once you are hip to how we women do that, you will hear it everywhere in casual conversation.

If you aren't feeling confident and authoritative, it's best to keep it brief. Don't let yourself ramble—say what you need to say and then stop talking.

2. Act like you know what you are doing.

Stand up straight, keep your hands at your sides, keep a serious look on your face, and don't try to lighten up the situation with humor.

3. Look like you know what you are doing.

Make sure you are professionally dressed in these kinds of situations. Acting with authority is seldom done with your thong showing. Look to most successful women, especially women in the public eye—like Katie Couric and Condoleezza Rice—and you'll find them in a power suit. While they might not hide their femininity, they don't flaunt it, either, in a Carmen Electra sort of way.

Practice all of the above in order to act with authority!

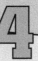

Counseling Services

Many of our boyfriends taught us things that benefited us emotionally and kept us from harm's way. If you desire more self-esteem, you need to learn how to feel daring and successful *without* a man. You might go along feeling brave when necessary and suddenly need to hightail your way out of dangerous circumstances, like when you're being fired upon.

Look at this section as your personal counselor. We'll show you not only how but where to meet the right man. And we'll help you discover your Boyfriend University "type." Your counselor is available and waiting!

How to Feel Daring and Successful without a Man

Jennifer loves to tell the story of the day that she and her dog, Big Guy, hit the open road for Mount Vernon, Washington, from Central California. She decided on a whim to traverse the same road that her father had driven on the family vacation every summer, but this time by herself. A daring move for a young woman! The trip, which she took for fun, took nineteen hours. All the hotels and motels at her destination in Mount Vernon were booked solid, so she convinced the manager at the last motel she tried to let her sleep in her car in the parking lot.

Jennifer considers it one of the best experiences of her life—sleeping in the car and all. "I had this revelation! I can do it. I don't need a man to go anywhere." Moreover, she felt this liberation of doing whatever she wanted to do on the open road. If she wanted to stop and see something, she would. "We'd always ask our parents to stop at Anderson's, famous for its thick split pea soup, and they never would. I stopped." There wasn't anyone to tell her that they had to keep driving, no one with whom to fight over music choices on the radio.

How does one feel daring and successful without a man? It's the whole premise of this book. Every lesson is meant to teach you how to do just that. The more self-assured and competent you are, we believe, the sexier and more successful you'll be, providing you the strength to strike out on your own and eschew the earlier generation's mantra: "Never do anything without a man!"

This idea of observing and learning from men isn't new. It's a mind-set. You have to commit to not being afraid of things that generationally might have been nurtured in you to fear. Lynne's mom wouldn't drive at night—even to the grocery store a block away—without Lynne's dad. Lynne doesn't possess that mind-set. Certainly, everyone needs to take precautions, but *not* to the detriment of fantastic experiences.

Did you know that women throughout time have always watched men closely, hoping to pick up a few of their secrets? Joséphine Bonaparte, Queen Elizabeth I, Queen Elizabeth II, and

Jacqueline Kennedy Onassis all looked to men in their lives for guidance and then took their political and cultural strengths as their own.

Look at any women's magazine and you're bound to find myriad articles on how to understand the male species. Turn on the Discovery Channel and you'll see scientists debate the intricate mating rituals of mammals.

As you've noticed, we've gone further than boyfriends to hone our daring and successful selves. We've looked to fathers, uncles, pals, and even our friends' experiences. One witty, comedic friend, Liz Allen, considers herself a literary geek with a touch of prima donna. She laughed outright when she realized that her ex-husband taught her not only how to buy the appropriate tools for each specific home maintenance job but also how to find her way from any major airport to the hotels and conference centers on business trips based upon traditional highway layouts, numbers, and letters. "He explained the tools to me like this," recalls Liz. "You wouldn't put just any moisturizer under your eyes, would you? I see you use the eye cream for the sensitive skin around your eyes. You never use the grainy scrub under the eyes. It's the same with tools—you buy the tool that works on the specific area." And voilà! Suddenly buying power tools didn't intimidate her anymore.

We're not the first women in history to recognize how anything from a few courses at Boyfriend University to a PhD can enhance women's lives. And there exist numerous heroines in novels and movies, as well as strong, modern celebrities upon whom you may model yourself. Just consider these examples:

- **Jacqueline Kennedy Onassis:** Perhaps JFK taught her a thing or two about Cuba, but certainly he was mesmerized by her ability to translate for him while on an official trip to France.

- **Angelina Jolie:** She's saving the world one child at a time. Her full lips, Lara Croft kick-ass ways, and security in her sensuality surely sealed the deal for America's heartthrob Brad Pitt. And her character in *Mr. & Mrs. Smith* made every girl desire to don high boots, lingerie, and long trench coats. You surely received the message loud and clear that Mrs. Smith probably taught Mr. Smith a few things in return for anything she learned from him!

- **The Empress Joséphine Bonaparte:** She earned her crown with the intelligence she brought to Napoléon's military strategy. How did she accomplish such greatness—and have him worshipping her sensuality? She listened. She kept her ears open and then studied. History tells that once Joséphine took an interest in politics, she learned quickly, and Napoléon consulted with her on crucial decisions

- **Scarlett O'Hara:** Rhett taught her to enjoy herself like a man. Her second husband, Frank, reluctantly taught her the lumber business. Her dad taught her self-reliance. Scarlett remains the epitome of a girl who used her Boyfriend University classes to her advantage.

- **Katie Couric:** She grabbed that anchor desk from a man by forging her way into the hard-question arena. Never fulfilled with fluff stories, Katie took the masculine anchorman approach to her *Today Show* role and added all her femininity, too. Ever notice she always shows a little leg? And she earned a desk historically reserved for a gruff-voiced, older gentleman.

- **Catherine Willows, *CSI* character:** Marge Helgenberger plays Willows on the tremendously popular *CSI*. Willows retains her femininity in a world of men without sacrificing tenacity or strength. Though not her boyfriend, Gil Grissom, her boss, leads her at times to clarity and understanding about the cases.

- **Evey Hammond,** *V for Vendetta* **character:** Natalie Portman portrayed the somewhat reluctant player in V's vigilante plan. Nevertheless, Evey learns from V and becomes an unlikely ally in the revolution.

- **Sydney Bristow,** *Alias* **character:** This role put Jennifer Garner on the map and led to a successful movie career beyond the series. But, alas, who mentored Sydney in her CIA duties and fighting skills? None other than Jack Bristow, Sydney's dad, also a CIA operative.

So did we answer how to be daring and successful without a man? Yes. Learn and dare yourself to do the things you want to do. It's really not about the man. It's about you and your self-confidence. You and your desires. Be strong and love life. That's how you *are* sexy, daring, and successful—without a man, without anyone.

How to React to Gunfire

Goodness knows we don't want anyone to ever be facing open gunfire, but getting away from a gunman is an important skill to possess. Lynne's brother, Matthew, served many years as a police officer before heading off into a career in the paramedical arena. Sure, when Matthew was younger, he played "cops" with paintball guns, but today he's encountered real dilemmas and weapons situations. If you're ever in the line of fire, according to Matthew, there are some steps you can take that can save your life. Thankfully, Lynne has never had to use this skill to save her own life, but she's pleased to have it in her database—just in case.

This is a short section, with information we hope you'll never need to use, but nevertheless, here is what to do if someone is shooting at you. If you just hear gunfire nearby, get down on the ground, but if you are the target, you need to get moving.

1. Run away from the gunfire in a zigzagging pattern. You're a moving target this way instead of a sitting duck.

2. Run until you can't hear the gunfire or can find adequate shelter. It's best to have run so far that you are no longer near the gunfire.

3. Find shelter.

4. Call for help.

How to Turn an Ex-Boyfriend into a Friend

Both Lynne and Jennifer admit that there are a few men with whom they've shared a romantic relationship that became a friendship. In particular, Lynne fondly remembers Randall. Her best friend from high school set her up with this transplanted East Coast, Ivy League hunk during her junior year in college. Lynne and Randall first met on St. Patrick's Day at a comedy club. Lynne remembers laughing so much that her green beer spurted from her nose! Embarrassing, right? But Randall loved it. Mostly, he loved it because Lynne was laughing more at his jokes than at the comedian's. They dated on and off for the next year. Certainly the passion existed, but when the romance ended, the friendship didn't. Their shared laughter kept the friendship fresh and lasting. Though Lynne rarely talks to Randall (long since moved to another state and married to a lovely lady, who probably knows how to drink and heartily hoot and guffaw at the same time), she does hear from him. While he lived in her town, she often shared meals with this former flame. In fact, she continued their friend-ship into her pregnancies. "I'll never forget the look on Randall's face when I showed up for lunch eight months pregnant!" Lynne says, laughing.

The worst part of a relationship is the breakup. We have expressed from the beginning that you've got to leave without bit-terness and ask yourself, "What did I learn?" Remember Boyfriend University's motto: I came, I dated, I conquered! We generally advocate that you keep walking and don't look back; it's just too difficult to permanently end it otherwise. You also cannot break some guy's heart and expect him to be your friend. How would you feel if your man trampled on your heart and then asked if you'd hang out with him just as a friend, maybe catch a movie? You'd hate it!

But special situations do arise when two people enjoy each other on many levels beyond the couple thing. It's not easy, but here is how to turn an ex-boyfriend into a platonic friend and transform the breakup into a positive experience.

TIME HEALS ALL

Alas, Culture Club's Boy George brought time into perspective with his classic 1980s tune "Time." So many other musicians (and poets) have philosophized about time's easing pain, helping the development of a relationship, and so much more. Essentially, it takes time to allow your relationship to develop into more of a friendship.

HOW MUCH DO YOU MISS HIM?

After some time has passed, do you miss the person on a purely platonic level? Or could you take him or leave him? You might find that after a couple of months, you rarely think about him.

Don't play the mind trick either and tell your friends you don't have those kinds of feelings anymore, when you really do and are using the "Let's work on our friendship now" ploy to get back together.

HOW TO KEEP THE FRIENDSHIP

A close pal of Lynne's says, "Girls expect the guy to entertain them. But what do they bring to the table that will make him want to stay friends after the breakup?" Essentially, he's got a point. If you want your ex as a friend, you've got to be a friend. Just as you're learning from him, teach him something. Show him who you are *outside* of the relationship. If you love art history, he'll feel your excitement when you talk about a Poussin or a Picasso. Your enthusiasm will most likely transfer to him. Sure, men like their egos stroked, their interests to be interesting to you. But they also can't talk to a dimwit without any hobbies outside of shopping. Our whole premise of this book is to empower women to grab hold of life with a can-do attitude. If we love being fascinated by men and learning their world, why wouldn't a guy want the same?

DON'T BE BORING

And yet another eighties band enters the pages of this book, the Pet Shop Boys. Their song "Being Boring" discusses how a couple avoids boring situations by choosing interesting activities and cultivating their own interests. It was a motto that Lynne and another, more permanent, beau held in their relationship. Lynne and Randall were never boring to each other. They exhausted each other with conversations on everything from Dickens to diction, from astronomy to geology, from drama to comedy. Another male friend of Lynne's explains it this way: "If a girl ever says she's bored, then she's boring, because I can always find something to do. Take a walk! Watch people! Go get a hobby! What do you enjoy?" If you enjoyed the intelligence and respected the activities of the other person, chances are much better you'll like hanging out with him again and he with you after the heat has cooled and you're no longer a couple.

GO EASY ON THE COMPLAINTS

If you do get together and try to go the friendship route, don't complain about a current boyfriend. Don't reminisce about how great it was with your ex and bash your new beau. Why? Because all that really means is that you clearly want to get back together with the ex-boyfriend.

THE FINAL WORD

Remember the couples' skates in junior high? A lovelorn soft-rock or hip-hop artist crooned while "Johnny" or "Billy" held your hand? One week it was Johnny, the next Billy. But neither Johnny nor Billy really cared, because they'd moved on, too. Yeah, you really cannot have a friendship with a former lover unless *you both* have moved on. If not, you run the risk of one of you clinging to old feelings. Things get messy from here. With time on your side, you'll move on. He'll move on. You'll meet up without any feelings "like that" for him. He won't have any feelings "like that" for you. You'll laugh, remembering that St. Patrick's Day you doubled up with laughter and spewed green beer from your nose onto his white shirt.

Perhaps that's the best advice of all about turning a breakup into a positive. You need to have laughed in your relationship with the person in order to feel joy in the transformation. (It doesn't hurt to show up for lunch eight months pregnant, either!)

How to Know If He's a Fixer-Upper and Worth Keeping

Who hasn't been with a man whom you look at through rose-colored glasses? All of his imperfections seem meaningless, because you know he possesses that one thing that no one else in your family seems to notice: potential! Lynne's been there. She believed in her former boyfriend Alek Voljovich. Some education, a few years of military training, and a wicked sense of humor—these were his assets that kept Lynne dating him for months. See what Lynne learned about dating the fixer-upper.

Is the guy a fixer-upper or a lemon? Does he have potential or is it time to leave? These are two big questions women often ask themselves. The answers depend on many things—is he a fixer-upper in the "dressing right" category or the "good behavior" category? Big difference in whether you can potentially fix the problem, ladies! What follows are key ideas to keep in mind if you need to decide whether the guy you're with might be Mr. Right (if you could only tap into his potential) or Mr. Wrong-Wrong-Wrong:

- Jennifer believes we can put most "keeper" men in two categories: the handyman who fixes stuff and the nonhandyman who pays for stuff to get fixed. If the guy is neither handy nor able to pay for anything, he's a lemon. Get rid of him. "Really, you're not going to be able to change him," says Jennifer. "There's no such thing, so what use do you have for him if he's not handy or able to pay for things to get fixed?"

- You need to decide the qualities in a man without which you cannot live. If your guy lacks these meaningful qualities, move on. *You* cannot change anyone's fundamental personality traits. If the guy is a cheater, chances are you cannot change this trait. It'll take his decision to change on his own and then possibly years of professional help. You can't help him with any addictions, for example. Cut him loose so he has the opportunity to hit rock bottom and receive help. Perhaps he just might want the help by then.

- If there are specific attributes that bother you, decide whether you're willing to compromise. For example, perhaps you can overlook his weekend Birkenstock wearing because you genuinely love everything about him and decide not to begrudge him his comfortable hippie shoes when the man wears Prada each day to the investment firm.

- Peter North, a good friend of Lynne's, gives an interesting perspective on why no woman should ever try to change a man in any way. "She is going to throw a whole lot of instruction at you, most of which won't sink in immediately. The part that will sink in only does so after the girl finally leaves—which then only works for the next girl. Do you really want to train your man for another woman?" Apparently, North had a girlfriend who didn't like his interrupting her. "I interrupted her too often, and she was probably right and worked on it patiently with me," recalls North. "Now I don't interrupt very often, but it's only now that she's gone!"

- Generally speaking, most guys feel that girlfriends are going to try to change something small about their behavior or attire. "We just expect it," says North. He says with him it's always the way the toilet paper rolls, under or over. "Each time I switch it for a girl, my next girlfriend is just as adamant that it rolls the other way," North says, laughing.

- So far, we've touched on clothing, repairs, and behaviors. But what about the guy who never seems to find employment?

"Any guy without a job," claims another guy friend of Lynne's, Robert, "is a loser. Lose him." The only exception is the scholar. If you're dating a guy in medical school, for example, you might want to keep him and look forward to the day he ends his residency. He has potential to earn, after all!

• Really, ladies, guys can evolve. But they'll evolve without your nagging about change. Small things? They don't really matter. Go ahead and try to get him to wear a certain label or teach him the basics of great wines (in this case, he's going to Girlfriend University). But don't expect to change any deficits or delinquent behaviors in any man—or any behaviors for that matter. We've said it before in this section, but it needs reinforcement: you can't change anyone. If you're even asking whether to let him go or keep him because of that elusive "potential," let him go. Move on. He is not worth keeping.

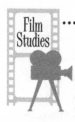

Film Studies

The character Tony Soprano of *The Sopranos* is a great example of how you can't change men. He's a hound who constantly cheats on his wife. She asks him to be "true," and he attempts it for a bit but ultimately goes back to his cheating ways. Even with professional help!

How to Know Your Boyfriend University Type: The Quiz

What type of guy do you gravitate toward? Take our handy-dandy quiz to find out where you should concentrate your Boyfriend University studies. These ten questions will provide you with a good idea of the kinds of men you seek out.

1. On a Sunday morning, you prefer to
   a) Nurse your hangover from the night before
   b) Meet with your Toastmasters pals
   c) Go to the new exhibition at the gallery on your street
   d) Slam a power drink and go for a two-mile run

2. You're staying at a hotel on a business trip. You ask the concierge to recommend someplace to eat. What restaurant recommendation most fits your preference?
   a) A Mexican restaurant with an extensive tequila bar
   b) A quiet, off-the-beaten path, Mediterranean place whose meals have several courses so you can linger over each dish and spend the night talking and eating
   c) A hip café, serving avant-garde food and providing a comprehensive wine list
   d) A raw food restaurant or a steak house—someplace where the food is simple and uncomplicated.

3. You get into a fight with your significant other. What do you do next?
   a) You get dressed up and go out with your girlfriends and forget about him
   b) You call him and talk it out
   c) He sends you ambiguous lyrics that you don't know whether they possess meaning or not
   d) You have make-up sex and worry about it later

4. You're shopping for a new house to live in. You like
   a) A high-rise in the city with all amenities within walking distance
   b) A spacious home with room for guests
   c) An old brownstone walk-up that can be decorated with friends' artwork
   d) A complex with a pool, a gym, and a common area

5. You're bringing him home to meet your family for the first time and you're worried that
   a) His lack of stability and immaturity will show
   b) He'll reveal too much and overanalyze your family
   c) He'll bore your family with his discussion of Mayan rituals and ceremonies
   d) He won't use discretion and will try to have a make-out session on the kitchen counter

6. You go to the video store to pick out several movies for the weekend. You tend to choose movies like
   a) *American Pie* and *Weekend at Bernie's*
   b) *Little Miss Sunshine* and anything Woody Allen
   c) Anything that won at the Cannes film festival (i.e., anything with subtitles)
   d) *9½ Weeks, Basic Instinct, Boogie Nights,* and *American Gigolo*

7. The two of you are going to a Halloween party and you want to dress as
   a) Tarzan and Jane
   b) Oprah and Dr. Phil
   c) Cleopatra and Mark Anthony
   d) Angelina Jolie and Brad Pitt

8. You're planning a vacation together and you choose
   a) An all-inclusive Bahamian resort where you both never have to leave the pool
   b) A couples' retreat where you deepen your relationship and communication skills
   c) Any city where you spend time exploring without the benefit of a tour guide
   d) A nude beach and spa experience

9. You meet up at a bookstore at the checkout counter. He's buying

   a) *Outside* magazine and the true-life adventure *Into Thin Air*
   b) *The 7 Habits of Highly Effective People*
   c) A biography of Jackson Pollack
   d) *Maxim, Muscle and Fitness*, and *Men's Health*

10. You see a guy at a bar. He's drinking
   a) The hundred-beer sample, and he's almost finished
   b) A martini
   c) Jameson, neat
   d) A Long Island iced tea

If you chose mostly (a), the type of guy you like falls into the "Spring Break and Summer Vacation" category (see chapter 10). He's a fun-loving, playful dude. Although he can be a bit immature, you'll always be doing something fun.

If you chose mostly (b), you go for the communicator type. You'd be wise to check out the lessons in "Communications Studies" (chapter 7).

If you chose mostly (c), your ideal man is either a sophisticated, artsy type or enamored of all things foreign. He's mysterious and interesting. Check out "Art and Cultural Studies" (chapter 6) as well as "Studying Abroad" (chapter 9).

If you chose mostly (d), you prefer a guy who is primal and likes sex, his body, and the physical nature of relationships. Check out the "Biology and Chemistry" (chapter 8) lessons first.

Where to Meet a Man, Particularly the Right Man

How do we possibly give one anecdote here? We can't. We've met wonderful men all over the world—literally! We do, however, possess a certain flair for finding them (and keeping them, if not forever, for a while). A few years ago, Lynne wrote a feature for the "Single in Sacramento" issue of *Sacramento* magazine. Charged with finding out the best places to meet men and the best pickup lines, she spent several evenings hitting all the hot spots. Dancing and drinking away these nights, she remembers only one guy. Why? Because when she asked him, tape recorder to his mouth, what he looked for in a woman, his response was, "You." She still smiles at the memory. The gentleman held a certain fascination for journalists and told Lynne, "You're the sexiest newsie I've ever seen." The guy knew what he liked (informed women) and went for it. You'll see in this chapter how we all should follow his lead when looking for Mr. Right. Go for what you like!

There are many ways to meet men, but meeting the right one takes skill. What follows are just a few of the best ways we've found to meet men we enjoy. And isn't that the key? If you're going to spend time dating someone, shouldn't he possess qualities that interest you and that you like?

Look around you first. We tend to go about our lives oblivious to the possible mates right around us, just within our scope. Lynne's grandmother met her longtime boyfriend by walking down her street, taking Lynne's then-toddler brother on a stroll. He lives just six houses away from her, and they have now been together for thirty years.

Is there anyone attractive at your place of worship, your bank, the grocery store, the shop where you have your car maintained, the police station up the street, your child's school, or your job? Lynne has met great guys at the market and while on a kindergarten field trip to the firehouse. Yes, firefighters are hot! Open yourself up to the people who are right there in your area. Do you have a favorite neighborhood coffee house? Lynne's sits three blocks from her home, and she has a whole group of great friends because of it. She hasn't dated anyone from there yet, but we'll see.

How about your job? Is there anyone in-house who interests you? Next time there's a meeting, look around. Besides being a journalist, Lynne also teaches. She's had dates with both a student's father (a former professional athlete on whom her best friend in high school had an intense crush) and her work colleagues. Tread lightly here, however, because your workplace might frown upon office romances.

Tell everyone you know that you're single and available. Ask if they have anyone they might set you up with. It's true that most people meet their mates through friends! Your friends know you; they can instantly weed out anyone who isn't well suited for you and send the good guys your way. Lynne met her ex-husband through his mother, Cynthia, who attended UC Davis with her. Okay, so the marriage didn't last, but they had beautiful children together and remain good friends.

Do something that's outside your comfort zone. You never know what you might enjoy or whom you might meet. Lynne and her friend Rhonda took a trip to Denver, Colorado, last year and signed up at the last minute for a risky, daylong white-water rafting trip with a guide. Donning wet suits, they both noticed the adorable "mountain man" who led their raft. While getting tossed in freezing waters and almost falling out on several occasions, they conversed with the guy, who invited them both to hang out with all the guides that evening for salsa dancing and Mexican food. Score! Lynne never saw herself with outdoorsy-type guys before, but this one turned out to be fabulous.

Figure out what kind of man you want and then learn where his type hangs out and what his hobbies might be. For example, let's say you've set your sights on a dashing, globe-trotting, rich man. Chances are the dashing, globe-trotting, rich man either flies his own plane or owns a private jet. Take flying lessons at an airport that caters to private jets. Or get a job somewhere within the airport where these men travel. Is learning to sail out of the question? No! Rich, dashing men and sailing are synonymous. Are you interested instead in a man who loves playing in nature? Learn to snowboard, rock climb, surf, or mountain bike. You'll find yourself surrounded by the kind of men you're attracted to.

Lynne possesses an unexplainable desire for Irish men and loves Celtic art and culture. She's thinking of either spending one afternoon a week in an Irish pub or vacationing this summer in Ireland or South Boston, an Irish enclave in the city. You must put yourself in the place where you're most likely to find the guy you're looking for. Ireland and Boston are both rich environments for Lynne to meet the Irishman of her dreams.

Jennifer met her husband by doing exactly this. She knew that she loved all things literary, especially words. "I love print," says Jennifer. Wouldn't anyone interested in words like Scrabble? While perusing a paper one day, Jennifer came across a personal ad where the guy expressed an affinity for Scrabble. On that alone, Jennifer answered the advertisement and met her husband, Peter. She clearly sought out a man who loved words, just as she does.

We believe so strongly that this is one of the greatest ways to meet the *right* man that we urge you to sit down right now and list all the attributes you desire in a man. Begin by looking at yourself and answering this question: What are my interests? Then ask, What do I want in a man? Once you have a list, brainstorm places you'd most likely find the guy. Are you a coffee lover? Hang out at cafés. Desire a dude who is rough and tumble, a cowboy? Kick it at every rodeo you find. In fact, learn to ride a bull or lasso a calf. You'll need to take these lessons at a ranch full of cowboys.

Go with your interests. We said this earlier, but the concept deserves another go-around. If you love gambling, go to the casino, honey. Wanted to work in the circus? Go to clown school. Have a fascination for the French? Then take French lessons and embark on a trip throughout France (or even Quebec, Canada) where you'll interact with many Frenchmen. Love jazz? Learn to play the jazz piano or hang out in smoky jazz clubs a few nights a week.

The key is this: You won't meet anyone sitting on your butt at home in front of the TV dreaming about going out. You have to *put* yourself in the position to meet someone who holds the same interests you do.

Do you really think you'll meet a lasting mate at a bar or a club? Probably not. The chance is pretty slim that there's one guy in there who has the same interests and desires that you do. Plus, clubs remain notorious as pickup-only joints. If you're serious about finding the right guy, follow the instructions we've given on placing yourself in the proximity of the type of men you know you'll like. But, hey, if you like dancing all night with a fruity drink in hand, go for it.

Try online dating. In our age, technology rules. There's a dating site for everyone. You needn't try only the big guys like Match.com and eHarmony.com. Dating sites exist on the World Wide Web for virtually every ethnicity and even fetish. Jennifer, remember, found her husband through the personals, so if you like piña coladas, let your online personal advertisement find the guy who likes getting caught in the rain!

No matter how you choose to find Mr. Right—through online dating, by begging friends to set you up, or by learning something new—do it with confidence. Virtually every boyfriend and guy friend (without benefits) attests to Lynne that confidence is the sexiest quality in a woman. Lack of confidence, on the other hand, will turn a guy off quickly. Just don't mistake confidence with ego.

Myriad books and Internet material provide ideas for the best places to meet men. Library shelves are filled with titles on relationships. Sit at your computer, log on to any search engine, and type "best places to meet men." You'll be amazed at the ideas. When Lynne wrote her article about where to meet guys, bookstores ranked high as a great place.

A final word: If you go against your own interests and personality, you'll find yourself sorely disappointed. If, for example, you lead a traditional Christian lifestyle, you won't want to accept a date with an atheist. But for the most part, finding men is pretty easy. Simply don't stay inside; go out and do something.

5

Leaving Home and Living on Your Own

When you go away to school, you need three important skills: (1) general knowledge of car mechanics, (2) how to make small repairs, and (3) general knowledge of the kitchen. It's pretty scary when your car breaks down. Isn't it a relief when you know what to do for your vehicle? Likewise, when you need to unclog a toilet or hang a picture, you can't call on Daddy! And what about cooking meat and making pastry? Both Lynne and Jennifer dated men with these handy skills—a way to get them home and a way to get them food. Just as it might prove a relief to know why your car isn't starting, likewise it's a relief when you know how to carve a turkey. Ever met a man who could cook? We have, and how we loved hanging out in the kitchen with them whenever we got the chance! Men who can cook are sexy. Men who can cook make good husbands. Men who can cook paid attention to their mothers. If a man can cook, it means all of these good things.

So what did we learn from men in the kitchen, the home, and

the garage? How to use knives, for one thing. Here are some others: How to Barbecue Anything, How to Make Killer Spaghetti Sauce, How to Guess Why Your Car Won't Start, How to Control a Skid, How to Properly Pound a Nail, and much more. These skills will last you a lifetime, so make sure you learn them now. Plus, you'll gain a huge sense of pride and independence when you don't have to call on a man for help.

How to Guess Why Your Car Won't Start

Jennifer and Lynne have both spent time around men who are somewhat car-focused. This can be a very handy thing indeed when it comes to figuring out your own car and why turning the key in the ignition isn't accomplishing anything. In fact, Jennifer spent so much time around race cars (mostly the kind of race cars that suddenly wouldn't start when the race was announced) with one boyfriend that she is still relieved to turn on her car and have it actually start. But if it doesn't, she has a hazy idea of what might be going on and how to deal with it.

When cars won't start there are usually just a few things you need to check. This may seem like a no-brainer, but first make sure the car is in park (many cars won't start otherwise).

If the car is in park, then check to see if the battery is dead. When you turn the key and nothing happens, try to turn on the headlights and see if they work. If they don't, there is a good chance you just have a dead battery. Call a tow truck or ask around for a jump-start. You can jump-start a car easily yourself; we have a lesson for that, too, later in the chapter. Beyond those simple things, there are some other quick fixes that might work. Here are the basics.

When you put air, gasoline, and a spark in close proximity to one another, an explosion results. This is the basic operating principle of every car ever built. Once running, the engine sucks air and gasoline into a confined space, lights it with a spark, and uses the explosion to push the car along (and suck in more air and gas). It's actually a very simple process, despite what Dwayne down at the Texaco station might have you believe.

So if your car won't start, it's missing one of those three things: air, gas, or a spark. The air problem is pretty easy to address—check your air filter and make sure it's not totally clogged. If you find prehistoric layers of dirt, crud, soot, dead bees . . . that sort of thing, then you probably need a new filter. While you've got it out, go ahead and try to start the car. If it runs, you've found the problem. Drive immediately to the nearest parts store or an oil-change place and get a new filter and put it in. Do not be tempted to drive around for weeks without an air filter, as this will lead to problems that cost real money to fix.

The gasoline problem is a little more complicated. Obviously, you've got gas in the car, right? Of course you do. Just to be sure, though, turn the car key to the ignition setting but don't try to start it. Check the gas gauge. If it moves away from the "E," even just a little, then there's probably gas in the tank, but that gas has to get to the engine. Moving gas from the tank to the engine is the job of the fuel pump, and if it's broken, you can't start the car.

If you have an older car with a carburetor, you can take the air filter off and take a sniff in the barrel of the carb. If you get a strong whiff of gasoline, then you're okay. If the air in the carb smells a lot like the air in the rest of the engine compartment, then you've probably got a bad fuel pump.

To check the fuel pump in a car with fuel injection instead of a carburetor (most all newer cars), you should get a friend to turn the key from off to ignition while you listen closely near the rear of the car for a high-pitched whine when the key is in the ignition position. That's the sound of the fuel pump running. The sound could be very faint, so try it a couple of times when you know the fuel pump is working (maybe today), so you know what to listen for. If the pump isn't working, you're pretty much stuck, unfortunately. Time to call the tow-truck guys.

Having an emergency kit in the car is always a good idea. Jennifer always keeps a corkscrew in her glove compartment for impromptu picnics, but other important things to keep in your car are the following:

Wooden matches or a lighter

An emergency flare

An adjustable wrench and a screwdriver

A whistle

A space blanket (a light-weight emergency blanket made of plastic and coated with a metallic reflecting agent) and a hand warmer

Finally, check for the spark. This is the part that, if it works, will impress all bystanders and earn you huge points as a Woman Who Knows a Thing or Two. Heck, even if it doesn't work, you'll get big points for just knowing what to check. Tell anyone watching that you learned it down at the racetrack.

The spark starts as a voltage in a part called the coil and is delivered through wires to the spark plugs, where the voltage causes a spark to jump across a very small gap. This is the spark that makes the gas burn and the car go. Between the coil and the spark plugs is the distributor, and the thing we want to check is the wire between the coil and the distributor, also known as the coil lead (rhymes with "seed").

The distributor is easy to find—it looks like an octopus, with five, seven, or nine wires attached to it. One of the wires on the distributor will be off by itself, and this is one that connects to the coil. Follow that wire and you'll see that the other end is connected to something that looks like a big soda can—that's the coil.

Disconnect the coil lead (the wire) at both ends: the distributor and the coil. Make sure you grip the lead by the rubber "boots" that are at the end of the lead and not the narrow part of the wire itself. Each end should pull off with a little effort and slight pop. Check inside each boot to make sure there's a clean piece of metal inside. If the metal is missing, rusted, or looks otherwise damaged, then you need to replace it. It might still work, though. Reconnect the lead to the distributor and the coil and press them down snugly. If the connection was loose, you may have fixed it. Go ahead and see if the car will start.

If you do all this and the car still doesn't start, then it's time to call in the pros. You've done all you can without help from a mechanic.

How to Control a Skid

It's inevitable. Most everyone will have to slam on his or her breaks during driving. Jennifer spun out on black ice at seventy miles an hour once and controlled the skid so she didn't end up in the guardrail. Everything she'd learned on the racetrack came back at that frightening moment, and it worked. It happened again a few years later when she had to drive sideways up an icy mountain in Utah with the car's back end skidding out (don't ask; it was safer than pulling over) in the midst of eighteen-wheelers. So, here are a few things she'd like to share:

- Avoid the chance that you'll need to control a skid by avoiding the risk of one. This means slow down, especially after a first rain. The initial rain of spring brings all the oil out into the road that's been piling up over the winter.

- In less-than-perfect conditions, double your following distance. Instead of three seconds between you and the car in front of you, go six seconds.

* In other words, watch the car in front of you pass an object or a sign and count one thousand one, one thousand two, and so on, until you pass the same object. If it's less than one thousand three by time you've passed the object, you're too close in *perfect road conditions.* If it's less than one thousand six in less than perfect road conditions, you're too close again.

The idea of keeping a car length between you and the vehicle in front of you isn't safe. Especially at freeway speeds, that distance of one car can be covered more quickly than your reaction time. You'll hit the car in front of you, before you have the reaction to even hit the brakes. Use the three-second rule instead.

Steps to Take to Control a Full Skid

1. Keep your wits about you.
2. If the rear end of the car starts sliding to the left, turn your steering wheel to the left. In other words, turn into the skid.
3. If the rear end of the car starts sliding to the right, turn your steering wheel to the right. Same thing—turn into the skid.
4. Regain control of the vehicle and relax. You just avoided an accident.

How to React If Your Car Has Antiskid or Antilock Brakes

1. Remember to slam your foot on the brake pedal, push hard, and leave it there until you stop. Do not pump the brake.
2. While slamming hard on the brakes, you should be able to steer the car if you must. The antilock braking system should allow you not to go into a drifting skid.
3. If you go into a skid before you've had the chance to slam on the brakes and activate the antilock system, treat it like a regular skid in a regular car.

How to Jump-Start a Car

Jennifer's knife-focused boyfriend did have an eye for gadgetry. One Valentine's Day he proudly presented her with a gift that will always be remembered in her romantic history—a set of jumper cables. And he gave them as a Valentine's gift because, he said, "I think sometimes women pretend to need a jump just to meet men, and I don't want you to ever need another man's help." Ahhh, such a sweetie. Or maybe not. In fact, what probably happened was that it was late in the day on Valentine's Day and he hadn't given her gift a thought. Stores were closed, and what can you pick up at a convenience store at that hour? You guessed it—jumper cables.

Don't buy one of those panty-waist battery charger things that plug into your car's lighter. You will be hanging around for hours waiting for it to charge. They are too small and not powerful enough. When jumping a car, size really does matter. You need the biggest, thickest copper wires you can find.

Having cables in your car is actually a really great idea, not only for your own use but for the rush of competence you'll feel someday when someone asks, "Do you have a set of jumper cables?"

They are cheap enough that if they get junky and dirty looking, toss them. You don't want grease or battery acid on your hands or clothes. Jennifer always keeps a rag and a package of travel wipes in her trunk to tidy up after roadside emergencies. Here's how to jump-start a car:

1. Open the hoods of both cars and find where the batteries are. Opening the hood on any car can be tricky nowadays. Look inside near the driver's seat and see if there is a handle to pull and release. On older cars you can run your

hands under the front of the hood and see if you can feel a release. Squat down and look up under the hood or peer through the grill.

2. Move the car that is running into position so that the cables will reach between the two batteries. This can be tricky depending on where the dead car is parked.

3. Make sure both cars are turned off. This shouldn't be hard, as one of them isn't running, but make sure to take the ignition key out of both, anyway. You don't want your hands anywhere near where various fans or hot engine parts are.

4. Examine the batteries in both cars carefully to find out where the positive and negative connectors are. Positive is sometimes covered in red and has a big plus sign. Brush off any snowy material, which is dried battery acid and could ruin your clothes.

5. Attach the positive cable to the positive connectors on both car batteries.

6. Attach the negative cable to the negative connector on the car giving the jump, but *not* on the car getting the jump. Instead, clip it onto the engine block.

7. Fire up the engine on the car that works and let it run for several minutes before trying the dead car. Nothing? Give it another few minutes and try again. Still nothing? Call the tow truck.

CAUTION

Don't hook up the negative cable to the negative battery terminal on the dead car because batteries produce hydrogen gas, which can explode with a spark. If you attach that end of the cable somewhere else, like to the engine block, then any potential spark will not be near the battery. You hope.

How to Drive a Full-Size Truck

You rarely see a woman rolling around in a full-size monster truck. Look at any advertisement for large trucks, and it's geared toward men. But that doesn't mean that as a woman you cannot drive a big truck with skill. In this case, Lynne's dad initially taught her how to maneuver a full-size, cargo-carrying vehicle while in college—but her skills were honed when she let Topher, a cowboy, enter her life. No respectable cowboy drives anything other than a Ford or a Chevy monster truck. Topher taught Lynne even more about staying safe and making room on the road when your vehicle takes up half of that road. Here's what you need to do:

1. Have patience when starting the engine. A truck engine might take a bit longer to start, because the engine is larger. Think of how quickly a mouse can scurry across the floor and then think of an elephant. The elephant will build speed, but it takes time for the momentum to kick in.

2. When turning corners, go wide. You make the corner wider than you normally would because of the length of the truck. You don't want the back end of your vehicle in the lane (and the car) next to yours.

3. When parking, make sure to have enough space to open your doors and exit. You may think that you fit only to find that no one can exit the vehicle.

4. Also when parking, start farther back and twist the car in at a wider angle, taking care not to sideswipe the other cars.

5. Always create an out for yourself in any parking situation. You never want to pull right up to the bumper, for example, of the car in front of you while parallel parking. A truck is

big! You'll need more space to get in and out of areas—even three-point turns.

6. Leave more room between you and other vehicles while driving as well—especially when braking. A full-size truck weighs more than a small sedan and will not stop as swiftly.

These are just the basic steps. To really become proficient in something like a big rig, you'll need one-on-one lessons. These steps, however, should help you maneuver a big truck easily and safely.

Now let's look at the minimum information you need to keep up a house. Lynne's mom used to say, "If a man can't be handsome, he should be handy." Okay, but how about not depending upon a man and being handy yourself?

How to Have the Basic Tools You Need to Fix Anything

Not only did Lynne's boyfriend Zack, the builder, teach her how to properly pound a nail, but he also taught her about the bare necessities that *everyone* needs in his or her home. One day when her curtain rod fell down, Zack came over to fix it. He incorrectly assumed that Lynne had the few necessary tools and hardware items everyone needs for upkeep and decorating. Zack drove Lynne to a home-improvement store and picked out everything she needed for simple home repairs. We suggest you do the same. Even if you don't learn to use all of them yourself, you can coerce some guy into teaching you.

What You Need to Fix Anything

- **Duct tape.** To quote Zack, "Duct tape can do anything—at least as a temporary fix and often as *the* fix." Need to make sure the hose from the wall to the washer stays put? Duct tape. Has the hose on your vacuum cracked, causing a lack of suction? Duct tape it! We recommend that the first thing you ask yourself with any necessary repair is, "Will duct tape fix this?"

- **Glue.** All kinds for all things. Always have these three: Krazy Glue, wood glue, and Elmer's.

- **Tape measure.** From hanging pictures to measuring the door to see if a piece of furniture will fit through to myriad other things, you'll need this one tool.

- **Lubricant (e. g., WD-40).** Does the door squeak? Is a knob sticking? All handymen have lubricant on hand.

- **Screwdrivers.** Get both a small and a large flat head and a small and a large Phillips.

- **Hammer.** So many uses for women when decorating!

- **Screw gun/drill.** Be careful and follow the instructions. This is a power tool. But it's the one power tool that'll do almost anything around the house, from hanging a picture frame to screwing a chair together to making a table. Make sure you buy the interchangeable drill bits, the pointed and often threaded cutting part of the drill, so you'll have the ability to drill different-size holes.

- **Washers.** Washer rings—flat, circular rings placed under the head of a bolt that serve as spacers or gaskets—are typically the easy fix on leaks and other things.

- **Nails and bolts.** You just need them.

Certainly, there are other things men have in their garages. But unless you plan on making cabinets and cutting tile, you really

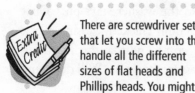

There are screwdriver sets that let you screw into the handle all the different sizes of flat heads and Phillips heads. You might want to invest in one of these kits, so you'll always have the right head to screw in anything.

don't need many power tools or supplies on hand. If you decide to get into refurbishing furniture and homes, you'll need a class or a complete book on the how-tos. For now, keep these items in your home for the fixes.

How to Properly Pound a Nail

This is an easy one, ladies. Ironically, most women hammer incorrectly. Lynne had a boyfriend once who actually helped his father build a home from the ground up. Rob grew up in the Sierra Nevada mountains, camping under the stars until he and his father completed enough of the house for them to move indoors. He taught Lynne how to hammer a nail, explaining that it's all about working smarter, not harder. Here's how it's done:

1. A hammer is designed specifically with a heavy head and a long handle, so your strength need not come into play. It's the action of your wrist and the heaviness of the end that propels the hammer toward the nail.

2. Hold the nail in place, fingers close to the end of the nail but firmly gripping it.

3. Most women grab the hammer closer to the head and try to drive in the nail with their strength. Instead, hold the hammer farther down the handle.

4. Flick your wrist to meet hammer head to nail. The hammer head is heavy for a reason. You'll feel less of the heaviness this way, use less energy, and drive the nail right in!

PUT YOUR KNOWLEDGE TO WORK

You typically don't want to pound a nail into a hollow area of the wall. Preferably, you want to find the stud. There are two ways to do this. The first is to use your ears: knock, knock, knock on the wall. You'll hear the difference between the hollow sound and the stud. The studs are usually about thirty-two inches apart. The easier way is to pick up a stud finder, about $5 at a hardware store. You run it against the wall and it lights up at the studs. Now you can hang that picture with the security that the nail is firmly in place! Another possibility to get all your nailing needs rocking? Find a construction stud to nail you, er, your nails into the wall or teach you how to do it yourself, preferably with his shirt off.

How to Fix a Clogged Toilet

What girl wouldn't have dated Paul "Pauly" Fortunato? Dark hair, blue eyes, and a sexy manner reminiscent of every role John Corbin has ever played. He steamed with an air of smart hunk! But the coup de grâce? He introduced himself to Lynne in a tiny Persian café by handing her a sketch he'd drawn—a profile of her sitting in the restaurant—pen on napkin! She melted. He was one intense artiste.

Interestingly, the skill this man taught Lynne was downright pedestrian. The son of a plumber, he knew a ton about toilets, including signs that your pot may be ready for a plugging, how to unplug a clogged toilet, and proper cleaning after a flood. She thinks she took Pauly aback when she asked if he'd show her the plumbing ropes, and one afternoon he gave Lynne a seminar in proper plumbing procedure.

Men pay attention to the operation of their toilet like they pay attention to the operation of their car because it's so central to their lives. How many sitcoms have you watched that poke fun at the propensity of the male in the household to spend time on the toilet? Since men pay attention to their "thrones," they're more inclined to notice any inconsistencies there.

Pauly said most men can tell something's amiss by the sound of the flush, the speed of the flush, the speed of the drain, whether the bowl refills at the right speed, and whether it refills all the way. These are all indications to a guy that his toilet may be off track and that a couple of quick plunges may be in order. The goal here is to avoid plunging a filled toilet. Men like to read on the toilet, not clean the toilet.

Signs Your Toilet May be Close to a Clog and What to Do about It

1. Pay attention to your toilet. Know its water levels and listen to its flush. Women are told to do monthly breast exams, right? We need to know what our breasts feel like in order to notice any inconsistencies. Take this same approach to your toilet, women. Get to know it.

2. At the sign of any potential problems, grab the plunger and a bucket.

3. If the toilet isn't already filled with water and clogged, fill the bucket about a quarter full with hot water, then add a small amount of clothing detergent and a splash of bleach.

4. Swiftly dump the water concoction in the toilet. Sometimes this is enough added water pressure to clear the clog. Flush again and see if your toilet works properly.

5. If nothing happens, take the plunger, center it over the drain hole in the toilet, and plunge forcefully. Wait for the plunger to retract. Plunge forcefully again. Repeat until the water runs down and you hear the clear flush.

Sometimes what seems like a simple clogged toilet may in fact be something far more serious—a plugged main sewer line. How do you know if it's a plug that you can unplug yourself or a sewer line backup or a broken main line that needs a professional plumber's attention? Pretty easy, actually. If water or sewage begins bubbling up through your tub or shower whenever you try to flush the toilet or run water in the home, you've got a sewer line problem. If water in any drain bubbles or drains slowly, you've got a main line problem. Finally, if all your own plunging efforts fail, you may have a foreign object stuck in there. (Parents of small children: Have you seen the cow from the plastic farm set recently?) First, call the city waste department and have them check the main line on the street. The city is usually responsible for anything that begins off your property but affects your home. Also, call the plumber. If the sewer line is plugged somewhere within the main line on your property, you're responsible. Pay the plumber and then disinfect the bathtub!

How to Unplug a Clogged Toilet

Ah, it happened anyway. Not to worry, Pauly taught Lynne what to do once the toilet did clog up. All you need are paper towels, a plunger, a bucket, a garbage bag, clothing detergent, bleach, and hot water. Once you have gathered up your tools, you are ready to plunge right in!

1. Prepare your environment. Put the hot water, detergent, and bleach in the bucket.

2. Place the plunger in the water-filled, soapy bucket.

3. Gather the other items you will need and enter the bathroom.

4. Assuming the plug-up is messy, you'll want to avoid having the plunger directly plunge any foreign elements. You can avoid this by taking the tip of the rubber plunger and circling

the water with the rim until any foreign substances within the bowl begin to move to the center and down toward the hole. You're trying to produce a mini–whirlpool effect here. If it works, great! If it doesn't, that's okay, too. You'll just be more apt to have a mess on your bathroom floor after the clog is cleared.

5. Next, firmly place the plunger centered over the drain hole in the toilet. Plunge slowly and rhythmically with force, waiting between plunges for the rubber plunger to fully retract.

6. If water begins moving and you can add some of the hot water and detergent, do so.

7. Begin plunging again.

8. Repeat the process until the toilet flushes freely.

PUT YOUR KNOWLEDGE TO WORK

Picture it: You're attending a cocktail party with numerous networking opportunities, and you're busy exchanging business cards and engaging in witty repartee. But somewhere between the pâté and the martini, you need to use the facilities. Imagine your horror when the toilet seems sluggish. Do you really want to bear the humiliation of telling your gracious hostess that you've plugged her toilet and paper is swimming to the rim, ready to flood all over her marble floor? Relax. First, wait for the water to stop running and try flushing again, holding the handle down until the water pushes through the bowl entirely. If the toilet keeps running after the flush, wiggle the handle. Usually this will drop the rubber plug within the porcelain tank, refilling it and stopping the run. If none of these tips work, see if there's a plunger somewhere in the bathroom and go to work. Finally, if all else fails, calmly tell your hostess that the loo is plugged.

How to Kick In a Door

How to kick in a door? Why on earth would you want to know that? And how did Jennifer and Lynne learn to do it? Ah, some things at Boyfriend University will remain forever mysterious. Let's just say it was a part of someone's government job to do this on a regular basis, and leave it at that. The fact is, how to kick in a door isn't a half-bad thing to know. It might come in handy someday. What if a small child has locked himself in the bathroom and won't come out? What if a romantic rival is cowering in the spare bedroom during a party, hoping you will leave so she can steal your man? Or what if you are the one trapped behind a locked door? Back up and kick, honey.

Knowing how to kick in a door will not only help you open a locked door, it will also help when you are called upon to buy a door yourself, or assess whether the door you have is good enough to keep you safe.

A door is such a substantial-looking thing, isn't it? So strong and solid. According to the folks who kick them down in the course of their workday, most doors really aren't all that strong and solid. Any ordinary residential door is vulnerable to a well-placed kick. Scary thought, isn't it?

To find the weak spot on a door, look just to the right of the door handle and go out about six inches toward the center. That's the weakest spot. Why? Because the part of the door with the lock in it may be strong, but kicking a few inches away from it will cause the wood to cave.

Step back far enough to give yourself room to kick. Lift up one leg, aim, ready, steady, kick. Kick as hard as you can from your center of gravity. Okay, then kick again if it didn't work. Fact is, in an emergency, you will probably have enough adrenaline to make this work no matter how weak or strong you are ordinarily.

Chances are you never will need to use the skill. But deep down inside you will know that you could if you had to, and that will make you walk a tiny bit prouder past all those wooden doors.

California Penal Code #844 authorizes law-enforcement officers to kick in a door under certain circumstances (if there's probable cause that a crime is being committed or if someone is in danger). So when a bunch of drug-enforcement guys are sitting around discussing their plans for the day, one might say "I'm going to go 844 a door." Has a certain ring to it, doesn't it? Just make sure that if you ever 844 a door, you have a damn good reason to do it; otherwise you will end up with a 415 on your hands (a public disturbance).

How to Make an Easy Pie

Jennifer is a big fan of pie and, lucky girl, has had more than one boyfriend who knows how to bake. Baking a cake is a handy enough skill; baking a pie is divine. So as to not hurt any one baker boy's feelings, Jennifer will daintily sidestep the issue of just who taught her the best crust technique. We'll just call him "Best in Crust."

A double-crust pie is lovely, but really, who has the time? Instead, Jennifer learned a simple technique for a sweet pastry dough that you can fill with just about anything. Leave the tiny bit of sugar out and you can make a meat pie, too. It has a fancy French name—galette—but you don't have to speak French to know how to make this easy mini-pie. Jennifer has already taught the simple technique to the next generation of men in her house. Her two young boys picked blackberries and made these tiny pies to sell to the neighbors to raise money for a go-cart. See, baking is a manly thing!

Knowing how to make a simple dessert greatly adds to your attractiveness as a guest. So get to work and learn how to make this one. It is a simple variation of a French pâte sucrée, or sweet pastry:

ℰ Easy As Pie ℐ

DOUGH

1 cup flour	5 tablespoons cold butter
1 tablespoon sugar	1 egg yolk
Zest of 1 lemon	3 tablespoons heavy cream

FRUIT FILLING

4 cups of fresh fruit (blackberries, blueberries, peaches, nectarines, raspberries, or apples)	2 tablespoons lemon juice
	2 tablespoons flour
	1/3 cup sugar

In a medium bowl, combine the flour, sugar, and lemon zest and then cut in the butter. (If you don't have pastry tools, not to worry. Jennifer uses two forks and works the butter in well and then uses her hands to smash it that last little bit.) Once the butter is well worked in, move on to the next step.

In a small bowl, whisk together the egg yolk and heavy cream and add that to the dough. Stir until the dough starts to form a ball and then use your hands again, darlings. Form the dough into a ball, wrap it in plastic wrap, and store it in the fridge for a good half hour. Once the dough is chilled, bring it out and put it on a floured board and roll it into a free-form round shape. It doesn't have to be perfect; this is a rustic tart we are making.

In a large bowl, combine the fruit, lemon juice, flour, and sugar. Let the mixture stand for at least 30 minutes to develop the flavors a bit.

Preheat the oven to 375 degrees Fahrenheit. Once you have created your free-form round shape with the dough, lift it off the board and put it on a plain baking sheet. Jennifer likes to use the kind with a raised edge in case the juices leak. Spoon the fruit filling into the center of the dough into a mound. Fold the sides of the dough inward, forming a nice tucked envelope edge around the fruit. The center of the tart will still be exposed, but don't worry about it. Dust the edges of the tart with a little extra sugar and some cinnamon if you like. Bake for about 30 minutes.

Voilà! You are now a pie baker, easy as that. To turn this into a savory meat pie, just leave out the lemon and sugar and use a filling of chopped meat, onion, garlic, and a veggie or two instead of the fruit.

Another easy thing to do with this same crust is to take a tart green apple, carve out the core, add a spoonful of jam or a dollop of fresh berries, sprinkle with liberal amounts of sugar, and then wrap the apple in the crust like a round little gift and bake. Too yummy, so simple.

Now that you know how to make a simple pie, why not try a simple flavored cream topping? The easiest way is to split a vanilla bean and scrap the seeds into the heavy cream container. Add the stripped bean pod into the cream also, close up the carton top, and leave it there for a few days. When you whip it, you will have a nicely scented vanilla-flavored cream for your pie. A nice foodie boyfriend taught Jennifer that simple trick and she still uses it.

How to Cut an Onion

Jennifer's only chef boyfriend kept late hours and would come home late at night ready to enjoy his favorite late-night snack— "Joe's Special," a simple scrambled egg dish created by a San Francisco restaurant in the 1950s. Made with eggs, spinach, onion, and ground beef, it always tasted wonderful late at night. He was happy to sit and watch Jennifer make it (her mother taught her the recipe), but sucked in his breath with disapproval the first time he watched her cut up onions. "Oh, fergawdsake, let me show you how to do that correctly," he said one night, then hopped off the stool and taught Jennifer a bit of knife technique he'd learned at chef school.

Knowing how to properly cut an onion is a kitchen skill everyone needs. An important underlying principle in cutting onions is to move quickly. The sooner you can finish the task, the greater the chances you won't end up with stinging eyes and tears streaming down your face. Not only should you move quickly, you should also focus on keeping it all together until the last minute. Keeping the onion together, that is, until that last final chop when you cut through everything.

An oddball fact is that wearing glasses or contact lenses seems to help cut down the stingy fumes. Both keep a bit of something between your eyeballs and the rising fumes. We don't recommend wearing sunglasses for this, but why not give your reading glasses a try? Here's how to do it:

1. Slice the onion in half, and working very quickly, peel off the skin until you get to the nonshiny, slippery layer underneath. Onions are not expensive, so don't waste valuable time trying to get to the perfect second layer; just peel off as much as you need.

2. Place one of the halves cut-side down, and cut off one of the root ends of the onion. Leave the other side alone, as this will hold the onion together while you slice.

3. Holding the root end firmly with one hand, use a sharp knife to make parallel cuts one way across the body of the onion, and then back across the other way to make the actual slice. Once you have cut both ways across the body, go ahead and cut off that root end to finish the job.

Here is another onion trick Jennifer learned. When you feel your eyes start to sting and water, stop what you are doing, run over to the kitchen sink, turn on the water, stick your head under the faucet, and take a long drink. Don't get a glass; just drink from the running stream. Why would this help stop the onion reaction? Who knows, but it does seem to clear the air of the onion fumes and give you something else to think about. Lynne's Albanian boyfriend suggests putting the onion in either cold water or the fridge for a while; it cuts down on the fumes, too.

How to Carve a Turkey

For years Jennifer sat at the holiday table watching the gleaming knife move back and forth, back and forth, slicing off a bit of succulent roast turkey with each graceful move.

It was like watching a beautifully choreographed ballet. First it was her grandfather with the knife, then her father, and now it's her husband. Such a manly skill, don't you think? Lynne, too, would be mesmerized as a child watching her father sharpen his knife before carving.

But there isn't always a man around when a bird needs to be sliced, is there? So you will need to know how to get the job done on your own, and we are here to help.

Before you cut into that turkey, this is what you need to do:

1. Leave it alone. That's right. Pull that bird out of the oven and then let it sit around for a bit. Give it at least twenty minutes before you begin to get it ready for the table. Carve it any sooner and the meat will be mush.

2. Snip off any string. If your turkey was trussed, now is the time to cut off the string and remove that little auto thermometer if your bird has one.

3. Remove the stuffing. With a large spoon, carefully remove as much of the stuffing as you can and put it into a serving bowl. With concerns about salmonella developing from stuffing left inside a turkey, you don't want to take the chance of poisoning your guests. In fact, it might just be best to bake your dressing separately in a casserole dish. Lynne actually removes the stuffing immediately after checking the bird with a baking thermometer. This way, she confidently knows the turkey is done. By removing the stuffing immediately, she mitigates her chances of germs breeding. You can easily find instructions for how to use a cooking thermometer in a cookbook or online.

Extra Credit

Turkeys need to sit around a bit after they come out of the oven, and so, too, do other roasted meats and poultry. Always let a roast sit for at least fifteen minutes after removing it from the oven. Not only does this allow the juices to reabsorb for a juicier piece of meat, but it also stabilizes the meat so that you can cut it more easily. Also know that meat still cooks while it is outside of the oven. For a rare roast, pull it out about ten degrees below what you are aiming for; the temperature will rise about ten degrees more while the meat is sitting on your sideboard.

Now that you've taken care of a few preliminary things, go ahead with the rest of the job:

1. Choose the right knife—a sharp carving knife with a pointed tip. A dull knife will slow you down and make your cuts sloppy. Sharpening a knife is pretty easy. All good knife sets come with an appliance that can be used both to sharpen the blade and to immobilize your meat so you can cut it without it's sliding all over the place. The sharpener usually looks like a mini-rounded sword. You run the blade quickly over the body of the rounded area. Instructions should come with the knife set. If your knife can slice through a piece of paper with little or no effort, it's sharp enough to use on your turkey.

2. Start with the legs and wings. Remove the drumsticks first by slicing in close to the body.

3. Slice the breast meat on an angle; stabilize the turkey with your fork while cutting vertically to create even slices.

4. Arrange the slices nicely on a platter and go delight your guests.

How to Slurp an Oyster

Jennifer and Lynne don't know many women who haven't had a man teach them how to eat something exotic. They've learned the finer points of eating everything from stinky cheese to sashimi. One of the untried items a man might offer you is oysters. The aphrodisiac aspect leads many men to order the sampler plate of oysters (usually twelve, paired in six for you each to try one from places as local as Vancouver, Canada, to as worldly as Namibia, South Africa). Indeed, true connoisseurs of the oyster know from where their favorite shell hails.

Lynne learned about oysters (and cheapskates) on her first (and only) date with Jackson. They landed at a seafood restaurant, and as she scanned the menu Lynne casually mentioned that she'd never eaten an oyster. Jackson replied that he'd been enjoying them for years and asked if she wanted to try some. "We should get the sampler," he said. After seeing the price, however, he said, "Gosh, they're really expensive, about two dollars more than in the South. I don't know if I want to pay that price."

He wasn't short on cash, and Lynne knew she was worth the extra two bucks. Thinking it was gauche that he made the comment after offering her the darn delicacy (which he nonetheless ended up ordering), she decided that this would be their first and last date. But the evening wasn't a total loss: she carefully studied his oyster-slurping technique and uses it to this day.

The lesson, ladies? Even on one date you can learn something. The boyfriend doesn't need to be your long-term man to offer a lesson or two. If an opportunity presents itself, grab it, and then walk away with more knowledge. Lynne did, and she loves oysters now.

Steps for Eating Oysters

1. Pick the oyster. You choose it by the location of its harvest. If you're new to the game, plan on a sampler. Make sure the

waiter advises you with a reference chart that shows where the oysters come from. Make note of the location of the one you find tasty. Then order from that region whenever you enjoy an oyster evening. But don't forget to try oysters from other areas again just in case you find another region's oyster that reigns supreme in your taste buds.

2. Decide on your condiment. Less is more. The fewer condiments slathered, the more you'll enjoy the rich flavor of the oyster. Lynne prefers a mere sprinkling of lemon. Some common choices to add to your oyster include hot sauce, horseradish, and cocktail sauce. Please don't mix them all up and drop a spoonful on the poor oyster—that will only ensure that you don't feel the texture or experience the taste. Rise to the occasion and try something new.

> The more horseradish, cocktail sauce, and hot sauce you drench your oyster in, the less you'll actually savor the flavor—and you'll appear crude. It's like covering a steak tartare in ketchup. A little horseradish or cocktail sauce, maybe—but a dressing? Never. And although many people do put the critters on a cracker instead of sucking them out of the shell, we don't advise it. Again, you'd just waste the taste and show your cretinous side.

3. Make sure that the oyster has been pulled away from the shell (shucked). Some restaurants provide the pull from the shell; others don't. Even if you're eating at a place nice enough to do all the work for you, make sure with a fork that the muscle is rolling around and detached. Otherwise you won't be able to do step four.

4. Place the oyster shell near your lips and suck the meat right

into your mouth. Use a little suction and that bad boy will slide right in.

5. Enjoy the slightly salty, flavorful delicacy.

That's it. It's pretty uncomplicated. Oysters are fun and sexy. Every girl needs to know how to savor one.

How to Barbecue Anything

Sometime during the evolution of men, their genes designated them as meat-a-holics. Men see barbecuing as an art—and no man more so than Lynne's dad, Michael. She didn't need a boyfriend for this skill. Her father is the Meat Master, the Grill Sergeant, the Paul Bunyan of Barbecuing, the Carnivore Captain! You get the idea. He prides himself on never transferring a lighting fluid aftertaste and pulling his meat off the grill at its juiciest prime.

> **CAUTION**
> Though Lynne's dad barbecued with a buzz cut and didn't need to worry about setting his mane on fire, ladies, you might want to pull your hair back when you barbecue. Burned hair is neither a cute look nor a sexy scent. But, to take a positive approach, burned hair does ward off insects. So if mosquitoes invade your backyard . . . not really. Pull your hair back into a ponytail.

Though Michael still uses the old tin-bucket-and-coal method, most people have upgraded to the propane tank grill. Working with propane might scare some women, so we'll give you the lowdown to safely get your meat on the grill.

You can purchase propane tanks at almost any store. Sorry, did I say any store? Please exclude clothing stores, shoe stores, or any other "womanly" stores. Your local grocery or hardware store should stock propane tanks.

Setting up the Barbecue

1. Lay a sheet of foil across the grill. Not only does it keep the food where it should be, but it also helps prevent having to scrub the barbecue.

2. Once you have your propane tank next to the barbecue, connect the tank with the hose that your barbecue should be equipped with.

3. When the tank and the barbecue are connected correctly, turn the knob at the top of the tank, just as you turn on a garden hose. Once you know the propane is running, turn on the barbecue. If a flame ignites, you're good to go. Otherwise, you will need to use a long-necked candle lighter. Don't whip out the ol' Zippo, as much as you want to. You may risk a serious burn.

4. If using a candle lighter, simply stick the neck into the grill and light the flame. Don't lower your face or any other part of your body too close; sometimes the fire may ignite in places other than the barbecue, so watch your hair and clothes.

5. When cooking time arrives, remember, marinating is key. Even the simple combination of olive oil, soy sauce, balsamic vinegar, and garlic can impress the most sophisticated dinner guests. Lynne rubs balsamic vinegar, a little olive oil, and fresh rosemary on tri-tips for a festive, Italian-themed grill.

Grillers begin by a hit-and-miss system of checking the meat. Once you've grilled several times, you actually get a feel for how long it takes to cook your meat the way you (and your guests) prefer—rare, medium rare, medium, medium well, well done.

6. Space your meat out on the grill. The thickness of the steak and how your guests like their meat cooked will determine how long you keep the meat grilling. True grill sergeants know to perpetually watch their food and remember how long it's been cooking. Lynne's dad cooks his meat in increments of four minutes. Usually, four minutes on each side produced rare steaks, his favorite.

CAUTION

Jennifer is leery of those propane grills, always flinching in anticipation of an explosion when she turns one on. So she has a little Weber grill that she prefers. Just buy those picnic-size bags of charcoal that actually are meant to be lit directly. What could be easier than lighting a bag?

How to Make Killer Spaghetti Sauce

Our friend Mary met a man with a sauce so good she married him. At least that is the story her husband, Tom, tells every time he proudly serves his spaghetti to a crowd of hungry friends. Did Mary ever try to actually learn how to make the sauce herself? No. Why should she when Tom does such a bang-up job? She's seen it done enough times, though, that she could do it if she had to. But you can learn directly from Tom.

This recipe will make enough for a dinner for two plus plenty of leftovers. It also makes exactly enough red sauce for a pan of

Extra Credit

So, if a man can make a good sauce, should you marry him? It is an awfully good sign that he would make a pretty good husband. Men who have taken the time to achieve mastery in anything, particularly something as useful as cooking, are a delight to behold. Jennifer's boyfriends who could cook were also pretty handy in other rooms of the house, if you catch our drift.

lasagna. Technically, it is a Bolognese sauce, or to be even more specific, a Salsiccia sauce, as it has as its base sweet Italian sausage. Tom also has a vegetarian version. Just omit the sausage and add lightly toasted fennel seeds (about 1 tablespoon) and 1 pound of diced cremini or portobello mushrooms sautéed in 2 tablespoons of olive oil.

❧ *Killer Spaghetti Sauce* ❧

1 pound sweet Italian sausage, whole or crumbled
6 cloves garlic, minced (feel free to use a heaping soup-spoonful of the jarred stuff)
2 (28-ounce) cans diced tomatoes (fire-roasted are fine, as are Italian style or whole—just dice them; this is not a recipe for fresh tomatoes)
1 cup dry white wine (preferably not chardonnay—use any wine you would drink, but do not use great wine)
1 small can anchovies
1 bay leaf
½ bunch fresh oregano sprigs
1 bunch fresh basil
Salt and pepper
Cayenne pepper

You can make this entire dish in two large pots: one for the pasta and one for the sauce.

In a large pot, brown the sausages on all sides over medium-high heat until there is very little pink left when one is sliced open (if using crumbled, sauté until all is browned). Add the garlic and sauté until fragrant, about 2 minutes. Add the tomatoes, wine, anchovies, and bay leaf. Stir well and scrape the bottom to incorporate the *fond* (tasty bits). Tie the oregano sprigs with twine and add to the pot. Chiffonade the basil (see the Extra Credit sidebar on page 85) and add it to the sauce.

Bring the sauce to simmer, then reduce the heat to low (there should be a few large *blurps* every 15 seconds or so). Stir often. Simmer the sauce for at least 5 minutes and up to a couple of hours—it only gets better with time. Stir as the spirit moves you. Taste often and add salt and pepper if needed or a dash of cayenne if you like a little spice. Remove the oregano and bay leaf before serving.

Another fast kitchen lesson from Tom— to chiffonade, pluck the leaves off the stalks, attempting to get no stems; stack the leaves a dozen or more deep; roll the leaves from one side to the other, making a loose coil; finally, slice the coil into very thin slices.

Tom also says, "Though my mother, who would not sweeten a sauce if a knife were held to her throat, would kill me for admitting this, sweet Italian sausage contains sugar. If you make any vegetarian version of this recipe, you may add up to 1 tablespoon of sugar without the risk of lightning's striking."

Variation 1: *Superfast Spaghetti Sauce*

Start your pasta water in a large pot. For the sauce, use the absolutely widest pan you own or can borrow. A large fry pan or, even better, a paella pan works fine. Omit the sausage. Add 2 tablespoons of olive oil to the pan over medium-high heat. Sauté the garlic for 2 minutes. (Just crush the garlic if you only have whole cloves: place the clove on the underside of a wide knife and smash the knife with your fist.) Add the tomatoes, anchovies, 1 teaspoon dried oregano, 1 tablespoon dried basil, and 1 teaspoon salt. Stir a lot—do not leave the stove for longer than a short kiss. The wide pan will reduce the sauce quickly.

Variation 2: *Mushroom-Free Vegetarian Sauce with Eggplant*
Eggplant can be a great substitute for meat. It is also a great sponge to soak up the sauce. To soften the eggplant without adding tons of oil, peel and dice 1 pound of eggplant (equivalent to 2 small ones) and sauté it in a pan coated with nonstick cooking spray. Stir constantly (no kissing). When the eggplant starts to soften and just begins to brown, continue with the original recipe from the point of adding the garlic. (You may also add toasted fennel seed to this recipe.)

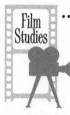

Film Studies

Men in the kitchen are so seductive. Truly a wonder to behold. And if you don't believe us, rush out now and rent the DVD for *Big Night*. Not only is it a wonder to watch Primo (Tony Shalhoub) working hard in the kitchen and Secondo (Stanley Tucci) working hard in bed (with Isabella Rossellini, no less), but you will stop the movie halfway through and go out to the store to buy ingredients for your own Big Night, we promise you. Sexy stuff.

How to Kill Your Own Food

There is a lovely old wooden boat somewhere in Washington, on whose deck Jennifer spent many a happy hour. What a nice boat. What a nice man. He didn't have much money, though (the motor yacht belonged to his parents, as it turned out), so she became quite handy with a crab ring so there would be something for dinner. Perhaps if the relationship has lasted longer she would also be able to teach you how to dig for clams, but no. That is all she knows—crab.

Knowing how to catch and kill your own food is a dying skill, so to speak. Anytime you have a chance to join someone who wants to teach you how to fish, how to hunt, or how to forage in the woods, say yes. In the meantime, here is Jennifer's lesson on crabbing:

Crabbing is not difficult. At a fishing store near the ocean buy one of the following:

1. A crabbing ring, if you are crabbing off a dock or a pier.

2. A crab trap, if you can go out in a boat and drop it in the ocean and leave it for a while.

In addition, you need a fair amount of line and a bait trap. You will also need the stinkiest bait you can find. Crabbers frequently share information about what is working the best— whether it is raw chicken parts chopped up and put into the bait trap, or hunks of old fish, or cat food, or maybe something left over from last night's dinner. You can also buy commercial things like "Smelly Jelly," which some folks swear attract crab. Jennifer isn't so sure.

Bait your bait trap, secure it inside to the bottom of your crab ring or crab trap, tie on the line, and drop it in the water. If you are crabbing with a ring from a dock, wait twenty minutes or so before yanking it up sharply all at once so that the sides close up and trap any crab inside. If you have a boat and are dropping crab traps down for a while, come back in a few hours, or the next day, according to the local laws about how long you can leave your traps out.

Pull up your crab traps and . . . wow! You caught one! But is it a boy or a girl? Most regulators allow you to keep only male crabs (what with the need to repopulate the species and all) and then only if they are over a certain size. In Washington,

CAUTION

Please check with your local fish and game department to learn what the regulations are and what licenses are required. The fines for illegal shellfish hunting can be steep. Acquaint yourself with the minimum sizes, and learn how to tell a male from a female.

where Jennifer still crabs (although on a much smaller boat), they have to be at least 6½ inches long.

Freshwater lakes and rivers can also be great sources of crawfish, sort of tiny little lobsters that you can catch the same way as crabs. Pick up a crawfish (or a crawdad, if you want to sound a bit country) trap at a fishing store, puncture a can of dog food, and stick it in the trap. Crawfish hibernate in the muddy banks during the winter, so do this in the spring or summer. You'll feel like such an outdoorswoman, we swear.

One of the rewarding things about having a useful skill is teaching it to someone else and watching him or her use it. Jennifer now stays on the beach and watches her young sons row out to check the crab traps a few times a day. She does drop them alive into a pot of boiling water (the crabs, not her sons), as her boys haven't yet grown into the cooking part of crabbing. Bring the water to a full boil, drop 'em in, and let them cook at a boil for a full twenty minutes. Check to make sure the crab is still alive before you drop it in, otherwise it will poison you when you eat it.

Now, on to the killing part. The first time, Jennifer held that live crab poised over the pot for the longest time, postponing the moment she would murder something. A sudden shudder of vegetarian tendencies erupted there in the kitchen. Why was she so hesitant? She eats meat. In fact, she loves meat. She has no illusions about what the life of a cow is like and how it ends up on her grill, juicy and sizzling. But she has never had to be the one to wield the gun or the butcher knife in order to get it there. At last her clenched fingers relaxed, dropping the crab to its watery fate. She covered the pot with a lid to keep the boil going, although it might also have been so that she didn't have to watch that desperate, waving claw reaching out of the water. Since then she's dropped crab after crab to its death in

Heading out to sea in search of big fish—now there is an intimidating vision. A big diesel boat, a lot of cut-up fish parts, tons of equipment, and those chairs that you need to be strapped into. What woman would climb onto a boat unless she knew what she was doing? That was Jennifer's thought when she stepped gingerly onto a Mexican fishing boat behind Cub Trujillo. Surprise, surprise, she quickly discovered the secret of deep-sea fishing charters—so manly looking, but the fact is, the crew does *everything* for you! So get your bottom up on that boat, honey, and don't worry about a thing. All you need to know about deep-sea fishing is to say "Sure" if anyone ever offers you the chance. Just don't forget the Dramamine if you're prone to seasickness or are not sure.

a hot bath. As fast as she can catch 'em, she cooks 'em. No qualms, just anticipation of another delicious meal that is doubly satisfying because she did it all herself.

So even though she isn't out in the woods with a shotgun or a rifle, she is now a teensy bit more sympathetic to the views and beliefs of the various hunters in her life.

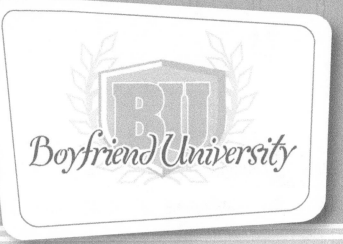

PART II

Finding Your Major

Everyone knows that once you arrive on campus, you must declare a major. Some schools might let you slide undeclared for a year, but eventually you need to pick an area of study that suits you. The chapters that follow provide disciplines that intrigue and guide. Have fun!

6

Art and Cultural Studies

So much of life is art, isn't it? Whether it is an actual piece of art, something you can touch and see and feel, or an artful way of behaving, art is a talent you need. Art appreciation, Lynne's and Jennifer's ability to appreciate (if not always approve of) the way their men behaved, was a valuable skill indeed. Whether it was the ability to watch and learn as one man used the art of bluffing and flattering to get what he wanted, or as another one artfully decorated his body, we watched and absorbed the lessons.

You remember (if you read Dickens, anyway) the infamous character the Artful Dodger. Many of the lessons in this section of *Boyfriend University* are ones we have learned about the art of getting through life without actually doing the work. Dodging the work, in fact. Giving the appearance of knowing something, or doing something, which in fact you do not know or have not done. So, by "art," do we actually mean BS? Well, sometimes. When Jennifer actually attended art classes

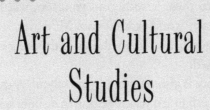

at Mills College (before she changed to a more useful major), she did notice a fair amount of bullshit involved in the art world. Pay attention to these lessons, and you, too, will be operating quite artfully in the world around you. Moreover, lessons on the more culturally sophisticated attributes of drinking cognac and whisky are addressed.

Creativity is also required in art school. A creative approach to what life has handed you is helpful in dealing with most situations, and we have learned from a number of men to be nimble on our feet. You, too, will soon think and act creatively when it comes to decorating your walls with awards, adapting a man's shirt for your own personal use, or developing ways to keep your relationship lively after the honeymoon phase has faded.

How to Have Fun

Our checkered dating history makes it sound as if neither of us ever kept a man around for long. Far from it—we both had long periods of being in a committed relationship, when we only went out with the same man. After a while, it's so easy to fall into a routine, to go to the same restaurants, the same sports events, hang out with the same friends. And that can all feel boring and stifling pretty quickly, can't it?

And then there was Jennifer's George. He had a way of cooking up the most surprising outings on the spur of the moment. A walk in the woods to search for pinecones and mushrooms? Why not? An afternoon at home with old black-and-white French films and several bottles of French wine? *Oui*.

Here are a few tricks she learned that will help you plan fun dates and keep your relationship lively.

Check out the newspaper for the town next to yours. What's

going on there this weekend that will take you to a whole new place? Could be a weird food festival or a premiere of a new musical work. Anytime you leave your own familiar environment for a new one it adds a tiny bit of newness and opens you up to possibilities.

Create your own holiday: something like National Red Wine Night or Take Your Boyfriend to Church Day. Yes, really. Lynne attends an Orthodox church, and bringing a new man to one of the services has always made for a lively afternoon. Use your imagination; you could create a holiday a week.

Celebrate a historic birthday. Jennifer's birthday, October 16, is the same as that of Oscar Wilde, the famed author of *The Picture of Dorian Gray*, and a famously flamboyant man. George surprised her with a complete set of Wilde's works and a night of heavy English food and wine. Perfect. Check out who shares your birthday or what happened on any particular day at www.scopesys.com/anyday.

Learn something new together. A language? A sport? Anything that you both undertake together, starting from scratch, will bust you out of your ordinary rut. Start training for a marathon (okay, maybe just a half marathon) together on the weekends, or learn to grow your own vegetables. Make sure it is something that neither of you knows much about so that you are both beginners; it isn't always as much fun if one of you is already an expert trying patiently to teach your partner what you know.

> **CAUTION**
> Sure, you need to keep your romantic life lively. But a word to the wise: don't let your man know you think life together has become dull and routine. No one likes to be told that he or she is boring. Avoid using the phrase "You bore me to tears, and unless we do something different for once, I'm going to scream!" Instead, focus on the positive: "It's time for a change! Let's try something we've never done before!" Get his hopes up with a promise like "I've got this wild idea about something new."

Go outside. Hike, bike, walk—there is always something out in nature to be found. Being outdoors exposes you to constantly changing conditions (weather, daylight, and so on) and constantly changing landscape that you can discuss, observe, or just silently meditate on. No doubt you've read those studies about how sexy the smell of sweat is. We have, and we take the time to get sweaty with our men as often as we can.

Add new people to the mix. No, we aren't suggesting a ménage, but it is true that having new people around you keeps things lively. Because you both act differently, perhaps in order to impress these new folks. Your jokes will be funnier, you will send each other fond looks more often, and it gives you the chance to see each other through a new set of eyes.

How to Mix a Martini

Mmmm . . . that new Bond is a very sexy guy, don't you think? Wouldn't you drink a martini if a tux-clad Daniel Craig brought one over to you at the bar? Jennifer would, but bear in mind that her nickname is "Gin," so she'd drink a martini if Vince Vaughn shambled over in an old T-shirt with an icy cold one in his hand.

A good martini isn't hard to mix. What is hard are all of those sweet fruity things bartenders keep adding to them in order to get women to drink more. So if you skip all of that fruit and blender stuff, the process is pretty straightforward.

CAUTION
Don't drink like a little girl. And never date (or marry) a man who drinks like a little girl. Learn to enjoy and appreciate the taste of liquor without having to disguise it behind fruity tastes or frozen textures. A sure sign of an immature mind is when you are holding a pastel drink. Oh, go ahead and have a Seabreeze if everyone else at the beach party is having one, but otherwise order a basic drink and skip the fluff.

Gin did learn about martinis from a man, but for once he wasn't a boyfriend. No, this is a skill she learned from her dad, George Basye.

Making martinis isn't rocket science, no matter what some bartenders and liquor companies want you to believe. You just need to understand a few critical martini terms.

Martini Terms

Dry. Very little (sometimes no) vermouth added. The relative dryness of a martini has to do with the ratio of gin or vodka to vermouth.

Up. Served in a martini glass with a stem. This is, of course, the classic and elegant look we are all aiming for as we perch at the bar with this glass in hand.

On the rocks. No need for fancy equipment, really, just gin, vermouth, ice, and a glass. Jennifer uses a two-ounce shot glass and pours 1½ shots over ice. Then she gives a quick pour of the vermouth bottle into her drink and moves on with her evening.

Shaken. Want to do the full Bond, then? You'll need a cocktail shaker and a traditional martini glass. Follow the same basic formula as above (1½ shots of gin, a teensy bit of vermouth), poured into an ice-filled shaker. Put the shaker top on, and shake. Jennifer shakes for a good ten seconds.

Added touches. These include olives, onions, or a lemon twist. Some drinkers like to double up on the olives or onions, adding a bit of food to their drink, we suppose.

If you have the time, we highly recommend reading the old James Bond books by Ian Fleming. They're delightful, sophisticated, and sexy. Buy them for boyfriends; they're a perfect gift to let someone know you think he is strong, sexy, and capable of fighting bad guys on your behalf. You will also soon learn that in the Bond books, 007 drinks a wider range of drinks than just martinis. Brandy and ginger ale comes up a fair amount, as does champagne. The actual cocktail from the first Bond book, *Casino Royale*, is more complicated than most: "Three measures of Gordon's, one of vodka, half a measure of Kina Lillet. Shake it very well until it's ice-cold, then add a large thin slice of lemon peel. Got it?" Bond then goes on to say, "This drink's my own invention. I'm going to patent it when I can think of a good name."

PUT YOUR KNOWLEDGE TO WORK

One way to make an impression on the job is to invent a cocktail. Even if you don't work in a bar, it still will make an impression on your boss. Make up a drink and name it after your boss or the business, then introduce it at a company mixer or social event. Jennifer invented her own personal martini, the GinSander. It's a summery dry martini on the rocks with a lemon twist and a small sprig of lavender floating on top.

How to Choose a Bottle of Bourbon

Some of your men might have moved on from single-malt Scotches to single-barrel bourbon. No longer moved by romantic advertising images of the Scottish highlands and peat moss, they now gravitate toward gruffer images of rough-hewn Kentucky. Don't worry, you can handle this drink, too. Jennifer's men did, and she has made the switch easily from admiring beautiful bottles of Scotch to admiring beautiful bottles of bourbon and even drinking a bit of it from time to time. With so many to choose from, you need to make sure the bottle you bring as a present is not met with scorn from a newly minted bourbon connoisseur.

Bourbon? How is that different from whiskey? It isn't. Bourbon is American whiskey. Got that? Here is a quick lesson in what is in your glass. All hard liquor is made by boiling the alcohol and aromatic essences out of a big tub of mush. The mush is water, yeast, and food for the yeast. The yeast eats the food and, well, produces alcohol as its by-product. We collect the

One of the best ways to drink bourbon is when the horses are running—the Kentucky Derby, of course. Grind fresh mint leaves together with sugar and some water. Pour this over cracked ice in a collins glass. Add bourbon and garnish with a sprig of mint. Set yourself down on the porch swing and listen to them june bugs, wouldja?

alcohol and the yeast dies—poisoned by its own waste. There's probably a big global warming metaphor in there, but we're drinking right now and can't be bothered. The yeast food is the primary difference in most liquors.

Here's what you feed your yeast if you want:

Scotch—wheat

Bourbon—corn

Vodka—potatoes

Rye—rye (we thought about trying to fool you on this one, but no)

Cognac—grapes

Rum—sugar cane and/or molasses

To qualify as American straight bourbon whiskey, it:

- Must contain at least 51 percent corn in the fermented grain mash. Most bourbons contain a considerably higher percentage of corn than 51 percent.

- Must be distilled at no more than 160 proof (80 percent alcohol).
- Must be aged for a minimum of two years, at no more than 125 proof, in new American white oak barrels that have been charred on the inside. Most bourbons are aged for at least four years.
- Must be bottled at a minimum of 80 proof.
- Must contain no added coloring or flavoring.

Bourbon makers will often release their product at something other than the "standard" proof level of 80 to 90 proof. In particular, if you see something called "Barrel Proof," you're looking at probably a 120-proof drink. Be very afraid. This stuff is flammable.

Jack Daniel's is often called bourbon, and it walks, talks, and tastes like bourbon, but it's not. Lem Motlow Distillers (the makers of Jack Daniel's) calls its product "Tennessee Sipping Whiskey." Who knew? Anyway, giving a bottle of JD as bourbon would be a faux pas when sober.

Single-barrel bourbon is what you will need to buy to impress. Always remember this general rule of snobbery: if there is only one of something, it is better. Wine made from one grape instead of a blend. A wool coat made from the wool of only one sheep.

Extra Credit

The way to make most men smile (the ones who aren't attending AA meetings, anyway) is to buy a small gift-size bottle of Johnny Walker Blue. It is the perfect stocking stuffer. At $250, the entire bottle is much too expensive, but the little bottles can be found in duty-free shops or specialty liquor stores for closer to $50. And it looks so lovely there is really no need to wrap it. Bear in mind that this is a blended Scotch, though, not a bourbon.

Bourbon aged in a single barrel. For single-barrel, we like Blanton's, and we especially like Jefferson's, from a small producer in Bardstown, Kentucky, where many bourbon distillers are based.

Many of the more expensive single-barrel bourbons come in very nice bottles that it would be a shame to toss out. Jennifer happily refills her fancy bourbon bottles with Jim Beam, a very good inexpensive bourbon.

How to Drink Cognac

Jennifer's cognac adviser was a dulcet-voiced musician and disc jockey named Robert Berenson. On many a foggy night in the San Francisco Bay Area, Robert would carefully select the right classic jazz (was it an Ornette Coleman night or perhaps a Zoot Sims evening?) and they would settle in on the couch with snifters of cognac.

Her first night of cognac on the couch was a disaster, though, as the strong fumes left her nose stinging and throat burning. It is also possible that she was unable to breathe at all for a short time. "Oh, here, baby," Robert crooned, "let me show you how to drink this stuff." And he did. She's used it to her advantage several times since then. In posh dining situations she has finessed the after-dinner-drink moment with aplomb, thanks to her cognac-drinking ease. And for those cozy nights at home, few things are as rewarding as a crystal tulip glass of old cognac, just the thing to sip by a fire. She might not have the twinkling lights of San Francisco outside the window any longer, but the rich smell of cognac always brings her back.

Learning to drink alcohol in the beginning was really a struggle, wasn't it? We're confident that at this point in your life you can quaff a beer, sip champagne, and breeze through gin and vodka.

Do the darker liquors concern you, though? The bourbons, the Scotches, the brandies? They do seem manly, the alcoholic equivalent of slipping into a rough wool sweater. Once you get used to how it feels, you can settle cozily into the warmth.

CHOOSE A COGNAC

Cognac, like Champagne, is a region in France. Technically, all cognacs are brandies. Brandy may be produced anywhere in the world, but cognac can only be produced in the Cognac region. The quality and age of cognac depend on how long it is left to age in an oak barrel. Cognac does not age in the bottle as wine does.

Cognac has its own special language of aging, one that Robert made sure Jennifer understood:

Many years ago Jennifer wowed a snobbish boyfriend by ordering a fifty-dollar glass of decades-old Armagnac. It was a dramatic gesture of sophistication and devil-may-care attitude (she was trying to match his own devilish attitude), and it made the point well. Armagnac is a type of brandy, from a different region than Cognac. If your dinner companion orders a cognac, you might up the stakes by asking the waiter if they have any Armagnac at the bar.

V.S. stands for "very special," and refers to cognac that is at least 2½ years old.

V.S.O.P. is "very superior old pale," cognac that is between 4½ and 6 years old.

Napoleon, or **X.O.** (for extra old) are cognacs that are older than 6½ years old. Many X.O.s are aged for twenty years or more before they are bottled.

Any real cognac is good. Jennifer is fond of Otard. Robert was a devotee of Hine. Rémy Martin seems to show up in a rap song or two. And you should choose whichever deep amber liquid appeals to you the most. Try a few different brands over the course of a few relaxed evenings at a top bar with a good selection. One cognac per evening, please; this is very strong stuff.

CHOOSE A GLASS

There is a bit of debate over which is better for cognac: the balloon-shaped glass, or the tulip shaped. The wide opening of the balloon glass lets the aroma go straight to the nose, concentrating the smell (and perhaps overwhelming the taste buds). Connoisseurs of the tulip shape believe that it allows the aroma to reveal itself more slowly.

Robert liked a warm glass, either swishing a bit of hot water in the empty glass and dumping it out before pouring the cognac, or balancing the cognac glass itself over a larger glass filled with warm water. Some restaurants will bring it to you this way. Don't be alarmed; just pick up your glass with confidence and rest it on its side over the other glass.

DRINK YOUR COGNAC

Okay, here is where it gets tricky. First you need to get accustomed to the smell. Lift the glass up to your nose (not too close, please; no higher than your bottom lip) and take a gentle sniff. A very gentle sniff. This is a pretty strong smell, and if you get hit with it right off the bat you might well spoil your chances of being able to take a drink at all. Once you get used to drinking cognac you will be able to lift the glass a bit closer to your nose (or put your nose down into the glass and sniff like the big boys), but you will need to work up to it slowly.

While a wineglass shouldn't be cupped in your hand, cognac is meant to be warmed a bit. Don't be afraid to cradle the bulb of the glass in your hands, as though the glass had no stem at all.

The biggest secret Jennifer learned from Mr. Berenson was this: don't breathe in as you try to drink. Either hold your breath as you drink, or breathe out as you sip your cognac. That way you won't get hit with a big shot of heavy fumes, which is what might leave you gasping and struggling for air.

PUT YOUR KNOWLEDGE TO WORK

Once you've mastered drinking cognac without losing your breath, how can you use this to your advantage? You can certainly order it with ease in a business setting (after dinner, not before, and only after the major issues of the deal have been settled), or you can bring it up as a metaphor when describing a situation. "When this agreement is finally reached, we can all savor the triumph like finely aged old cognac."

How to Bluff and Flatter

A lot of what Jennifer learned from various boyfriends was that regardless of whether you actually know what you are doing, you should plunge in and give it a try. And then bluff your way through if you need to. Never admit your ignorance or expose your knowledge gaps.

Here's a great example: many years ago at a swanky garden party, Jennifer overheard some posh older man ask her slacker boyfriend if he could play polo. He shrugged and simply said, "Sorry, I'm left-handed." See, polo is always played with the mallet in your right hand. Unless you mount two teams made up of left-handed players, it is too dangerous for both horses and players to have a lefty on the field. The truth was, he could barely ride. But he never had to reveal that, did he? No, he took his gin and tonic, nodded politely at the old polo player, and moved off to join the conversation with a less horsey group.

When using this technique, you need to be careful and not overdo it. The best way to bluff and flatter is to say one thing quickly and then shut up. Don't go on with some imaginary tale that will only make your listener wonder if you are full of it. Just like Jennifer's nonriding boyfriend, just say one thing and move on.

If you are going to bluff in a situation, keep these pointers in mind:

1. Look the person in the eye.

2. Speak with confidence.

3. Say whatever comes to mind.

4. Smile and be quiet.

For instance, don't know anything about wine? Why let that hold you back from asking for the wine list with great confidence? Study it quietly, maybe squint your eyes and cock your head as though you are really considering a number of difficult choices Then shrug and say to the waiter, "You drink from this wine list more often than I do; what would you suggest?" Sit back and watch what kind of superb service you will get from that point on. Rather than think you are a wine dummy, the waiter will be flattered that you've pretended he can afford the prices and will happily steer you toward something he himself has always dreamed of ordering. Another useful line in this situation is, "If you were celebrating a birthday [anniversary, promotion, holiday, whatever], what would you choose?" Got it? Bluff by never revealing that you don't know one thing about wine, and flatter the waiter by asking his opinion. Works every time.

Remember never to bluff in a snide and mean way, but always to bluff in a way that makes someone else look good. He or she will appreciate it and give you whatever you need.

Bluff and flatter your way into great restaurant service: "I think you were my waiter the last time I was here. It was such a good meal, and you were amazing." Now, really, is that going to smooth the way to a perfect evening or what?

Bluff and flatter your way into great service in some snooty boutique: "Is this your shop? You have wonderful taste!" Say that to any snippy woman standing behind a cash register working for a small hourly wage and she will want to be your new best friend.

Bluff and flatter your way into an upgraded hotel room or airline seat: "You look like you are in the mood to upgrade someone! I will selflessly volunteer."

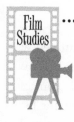

Film Studies

Con artists are always fun to watch on screen. So while we once again remind you that we only want you to bluff and flatter, not con, there might be a tip or two you can pick up from watching the old classics *Paper Moon*, *The Sting*, and *Dirty Rotten Scoundrels*. The sly smiles that actors like Ryan O'Neal, Michael Caine, and Paul Newman can conjure up are priceless.

So, will you need to bluff and flatter in your relationships? Heavens, yes. Although, bless their hearts, men seldom notice that you are bluffing and flattering. They will happily believe you are confident in their abilities and rely on their knowledge and are deeply, deeply interested in all of their hobbies.

How to Make Any Gift Fraught with Meaning

It will happen to you. Someday you will look up at the calendar and say, "Oh hell, I forgot to shop for Mr. X's birthday." Or your anniversary. Never fear, there are ways to pick up anything at all and make it terribly fraught with meaning.

One guy had a habit of giving Jennifer knives. How weird is that? Every time, he managed to make Jennifer feel as though he'd looked for the perfect gift all afternoon long and finally, finally decided that the best thing to give her was . . . a chef's knife to cut onions. A teeny Swiss Army knife to put on her keychain. A diving knife that was so long that when she strapped it on it stretched from her ankle to her knee. Jennifer did use that one deep down in Monterey Bay on a night dive to cut herself free after she'd become tangled underwater in some fishing line, so maybe he was onto something after all.

It has happened to you, too, hasn't it? The arrival of some off-beat gift that you know, you just know, he bought on his way to your house but hopes that you will see the great thought and planning in. How do guys do it? It's easy, really. You just need to know what to say.

Okay, here is the line you will practice: "I bought this for you." That was easy, wasn't it? And it usually does the trick just fine, without much explanation. Why? Because we all like to believe

Picasso seduced one of his many mistresses with what must have been the all-time greatest impromptu gift. He appeared at her door in the midst of a rainstorm soaking wet, holding a gift of a tiny and equally wet kitten. Awww. See how this works? We'll bet he said, "I got this for you. Didn't you tell me you liked kittens?"

that our love is thinking of us, regardless of whether or not it is true.

"Didn't you tell me you liked X?" You melted, didn't you? He was thinking about me? He was listening? So here is what you do next time you need to quickly come up with a gift. Just grab something off the store shelf and smile and say, "Didn't you tell me you liked fleece sweatshirts/diet soda/black-and-white films starring Sophia Loren/leather riding boots?" Go ahead, pull anything out of a grocery bag, hold it out to him, and say, "I bought this for you."

"I bought X, and I thought you needed one, too." This is a great way to cover up a shopping spree. Buy yourself a fleece sweatshirt/a diet soda/a black-and-white film starring Sophia Loren/leather riding boots and then get the same thing for him, too. It will make you look thoughtful and caring. George Bingham arrived at Jennifer's house late one rainy afternoon with a big bottle of single-malt Scotch and a handful of cigars. Could be he'd had a tough day at the office and was thinking of his own needs and interests, but when he set them down on the coffee table he said, "You need to know more about these two things and I want to be the one to teach you." Now that, you must agree, is an amazingly good line. Make it your own. At that point in her life Jennifer already knew plenty about both Scotch and cigars, but she kept that information to herself and allowed him to hold forth. It was a pleasant afternoon indeed.

How to Wear Men's Clothing (and Why You Should)

Sunday morning, and whatever shall you wear today? Why not pull on this comfy sweatshirt here? And these floppy pants? After all, they are lying right here next to the bed so you can just reach

CAUTION
Does he like you
to wear his clothes? It
wouldn't be a bad idea to
ask, because if it ticks him off,
then you should probably stay
out of his closet. Don't be hurt
if he feels this way; you don't
always like to share your
clothes, now, either,
do you?

down and grab them. Why wear men's clothing? Because sometimes, it's so darned close at hand.

But seriously, is there a better way to feel as though you've suddenly lost five pounds? We don't think so. And it's truly strange, but a woman sometimes feels even more womanly when she is wearing her man's big shirt. Are we right? You'll never want to give it back. Jennifer wore Cub's striped purple shirt for many years past the end of the relationship and still wishes she hadn't given it to charity.

Not all men's clothing lends itself to a woman's body. Here are a few style rules to consider:

- Men's T-shirts are never flattering to women. Cut off the sleeves and then pull it all out in a knot in the front—very sexy when worn over your bathing suit this way.

- Dress shirts are wonderful to sleep in, fun to throw on over a pair of skinny jeans, and great to tie around your waist; even cooler if the shirt has French cuffs and you have added the links.

- Tux shirts are not always flattering to a woman's figure, but if you are thin enough, try one with studs and cuff links worn with a velvet skirt or pants.

- Ties work best as a belt with your khakis at the beach only; you'll look stupid in town.

- Clunky men's jewelry looks great on gals! Jennifer loves the big clunky silver chain-link bracelet she shook down George for. Doesn't hurt that it's from Tiffany.

- Belts, especially big leather ones, can be hung loose around your dress. And if your boy is really, really big, maybe you can wrap it around twice!

Once you get in the habit, you might find yourself wandering over to the men's racks in department stores to check out the goods. Why not? Have items cut down or tailored to fit, and you will be charged less at the dry cleaner than you would be if you dropped off a woman's blouse! It's true, ladies. Goodness knows why we pay more to have our blouses dry cleaned (perhaps it's because of the fabric?) than men do for their shirts, but we do.

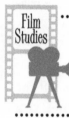

Film Studies

The all-time best example of how funky cool women can look wearing menswear is, of course, from Woody Allen's movie *Annie Hall*. We've never been able to pull of the man's hat look like Diane Keaton does, but hey, maybe you can. First you'll have to find a man who owns a hat, though . . .

THE ART OF TYING A TIE ON YOURSELF

The knot we're about to explain is infamously known as the Pratt knot or the Shelby knot, and here's how it's done:

1. Drape the tie around your neck, the wider end on the left and the skinny end on the right. The seam will face up, and you should be able to see a tag on the wider end of the tie. This is when you determine how long the tie will be. We recommend pulling the wide end past your crotch; think Tarzan's loincloth.

2. Once it's at the appropriate length, cross the skinny side over the wide side. Make sure to have the cross closer to your neck than your chest.

3. Now, holding the cross in place, take the wide end and flip it toward you through the opening between the cross and your chin. Once you pull it through the hole, the seam should still be facing up. Your knot has almost formed.

4. This is the tricky part. Keeping the skinny end straight, as if it's an arrow pointing to the ground, wrap the wide side over the knot (to the left). Once it's on the left of the skinny side, bring it under the knot and up through the opening between the knot and your neck.

5. Lost yet? By now, it should look as if the wide end is on top of the skinny end as well as the knot, with the wide side's seam underneath and the skinny side's seam facing up.

6. Lifting up the wide side, tuck the end of the wide side through the knot and pull, adjusting the length of the tie and the width around your neck.

How to Procrastinate

Ah, how very easy it is to procrastinate. Some folks, including some men we dated, never realized that they were procrastinating at all, but instead thought that they were merely using their time wisely. Procrastination truly is an art form, and both of us have learned from the masters how to incorporate it into our lives.

Have something that needs to be done? Not to worry; you must pull back from your eagerness and excitement to finish it. Instead, find something to occupy your attention. Make a phone call, go out for a six-pack, or see what's on TV. Distract yourself effectively and you are less likely to think about all those things that need to be done. Keep this up for several hours. Uh-oh, time for bed. But wasn't there something else you were supposed to have done first? Push that thought from your head. You must resist the urge; after all, you were just headed off to bed and shouldn't let yourself be distracted this late at night. What's that you say? The project is now due and you haven't done it? Relax, take a deep breath, and think about breakfast.

Okay, now make it happen. We know you do your best work under pressure, don't you?

How to Fake Your Way to a Clean House

Early in Jennifer's relationship with Cub Trujillo, he lived with his brother and another friend. They were just out of high school, and she was . . . well, she was already a few years out of high school. A year or so out of college, in fact, but who's counting? (Read How to Feign Interest in a Much Younger Date in chapter 7.) Sweet boy, he acted as if his mom were on her way, rushing around behind the closed door while Jennifer waited patiently in the hall (her apartment was one floor above theirs) listening to the sounds of young Cub stashing things under the bed to make the place look neater.

We've all had those days. Okay, maybe we haven't all had those days when we were dating young boys, but we've all had those days when we never got around to making the bed or putting the dishes away. Then comes a knock at the front door, and pandemonium breaks out. Not to worry;

The key to making visitors think your house is clean is to have it smell good. So invest in scented candles for the bathroom, a pot of potpourri for the living room, a big bouquet of gardenias from your garden in your bedroom, freshly picked rosemary in a jar for your kitchen. Keep their noses working and they will never notice the sloppy bits.

you can make your house look as neat as Cubby did for his older woman, Jennifer.

Stashing everything under the bed is a good first step. And the best kinds of beds have dust ruffles around them so that you can't see what (or who, if it comes to that) is hiding underneath.

It is also vitally important that you keep a lot of empty grocery bags on hand, both the paper and the plastic kind. Paper grocery bags are wonderful for storing paperwork and files and magazines and the mail that has piled up for the past few weeks. Just scoop up all that stuff, put it in the bag, and stash it in a closet if there's no more room under your bed. Jamming all of that stuff into a plastic bag is a bit messier; to properly stash your paper stuff you need stiffer bag sides, you see. Always keep your big department store shopping bags on hand, too. In a pinch you can jam everything in there and smash some tissue paper on top and leave them lined up in a corner. Your guests will think you've just come home from a round of shoe shopping.

Plastic bags are what you need for any overflowing trash cans or smelly stuff that needs to go out of the kitchen pronto so that it can air out before your friends arrive. Give your sinks and toilets a quick spray of cleaner and wipe of a towel, even if you don't have a chance to actually scour them.

Look around on the floor. If you don't have time to bring out the vacuum, are there big pieces of toast or the lost top from a water bottle that you can pick up?

CAUTION

Under no circumstances should you put your smelly wet sponge in the microwave just before guests arrive. Yes, at some point you should try to kill the germs in it, but understand that the smell of cooked mold is not appealing, and save it for some day when you are not having people over. Instead, toss the sponge in the washing machine or dishwasher (making sure you run the dishwasher prior to your guests' arrival). Or just toss the sponge; it's relatively cheap to replace.

The final touch is to rub lemony furniture polish on top of all exposed wood surfaces. The backs of chairs is a great place to give a quick dust to; anyone sitting in the chair a few minutes later will be convinced that your cleaning lady just left.

An important trait to absorb from *Boyfriend University* is to not obsess over the cleanliness of your house. Chances are it is really just fine and no one will notice anything amiss. Close your eyes and picture the last time you dropped in on a friend. Can you picture what her carpet looked like? Or if there was laundry on the kitchen table? No? We didn't think so. So let go and don't worry about what your friends will be looking at when they visit you. A quick word of warning, though, about another little something Jennifer learned from watching Cub. Don't hide your dirty socks behind your pillows; guests will surely find them.

PUT YOUR KNOWLEDGE TO WORK

Does a messy desk equal a messy mind? Some bosses do seem to believe that, so be prepared to use this same cleaning technique when you get wind of a surprise visit. Have those shopping bags and tissue paper ready to scoop the mess off your desk and cover it up quickly.

How to Talk about Wine without Knowing a Thing about It

One of Jennifer's least sophisticated moments involves wine. While in the company of a handsome prince (yes, a real prince, but the less said about that college romance, the better) she revealed herself as a total wine rube in front of a dinner table full of guests.

After draining a glass of expensive French wine, she held her glass up and loudly said, "Ewww, look, it has mud at the bottom!" Heads turned her way, and the prince blushed with embarrassment at his date's dumb faux pas. Any oenophile would have known that was sediment from the bottle.

With more than a few years of perspective on this incident, Jennifer can now laugh about it. The fact remains that much of the wine world takes itself way, way too seriously. We advise you not to get caught up in it all. Another wine aficionado boyfriend of Jennifer's, Jivan, the buyer for a large national chain, told her to always relax and enjoy what is in the glass in front of you. Learn what you like, and don't let anyone make you feel stupid. Please don't say, "Ewww, look at the mud in my glass!" but other than that, don't sweat it too much.

Stuck at the table with a few wine snobs? Here is how to handle the situation.

If it is your turn to order the wine, steer away from ones with cutesy and silly labels, the kind with animals or cars on them. Plain labels are almost always found on good wine. Understand that those other companies are trying to get you—and women in general—

Extra Credit

When wine tasting, you must spit. If you keep swallowing, you will become inebriated. Once impaired, you probably won't be able to tell anything about the wine (or about anything else, for that matter). So, really, you must spit. Jennifer once found herself on a barrel-tasting tour with a group of professionals (a wine industry professional, she is not). So she had to spit, which was not a skill she started out with that afternoon. By the end of the day, with the help of a few sympathetic men, she could. We know it is hard, so why not practice a few times in the shower. Fill your mouth with a small sip of water, swish it around a bit, and then try to spit nice and neatly toward whatever spot in the shower you want.

to buy their mediocre wine. Don't let them win. Order a wine from an old French vineyard and you will get a better glass of wine. And feel free to loudly trumpet the fact that you avoided falling into that obvious consumer trap. See, you look like a wine sophisticate already!

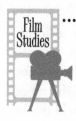

Film Studies

Get ready to taste wine by watching the wonderful independent film *Sideways*. By the end of it you will be convinced that merlot is a scourge upon the world, but try to ignore the feeling and order a glass of it anyway anytime you want. Still don't feel confident enough to taste and talk wine? Review our earlier lesson on How to Bluff and Flatter.

If you are worried about ordering the wrong thing in a restaurant in front of friends or colleagues, then bring your own. Another wine boyfriend let Jennifer in on the formula for pricing wine in restaurants, and it is a shocking 200 percent markup. So always be leery of the least expensive bottles on the list; you can probably pick those up at the grocery store for under $10. Instead, go ahead and appear knowledgeable by spending an afternoon in a friendly wine shop with an owner who will help you choose a good bottle to bring to the occasion, and then pay a "corkage" fee, the $10 or so that a restaurant charges when you bring your own wine. The restaurant deserves to make money, too.

Wine was meant to accompany food—don't lose track of that. In fact, some folks think of it as a type of food and consider a meal incomplete without it.

Yes, there might be sediment at the bottom of your glass, but it probably isn't dirt. Older wines have a tendency to develop sediment, so chances are you should smile and enjoy what you've been poured. You could also say with a knowing tone, "Oooh, sediment. Lovely."

Don't be distracted by the fuss nowadays about wineglasses. Buy two Reidels if you want to impress. All other wineglasses should come from Target, as your crystal will always break. Again, with a table of snobs, just complain about how much money you've wasted on broken crystal and that you decided long ago to spend your money on the wine instead of the glass. That ought to distract them.

And always remember Jivan's advice to Jennifer: relax and enjoy what's in your glass. There's no reason to be afraid of wine. Try everything from a cheap bottle to an expensive one. When you come across something you love, you will know it instantly. And then you will have it—your favorite wine of all time. Something for you to talk about when the wine talk starts up.

How to Win an Award

Ever gone into an office and been dazzled by the various plaques and awards displayed on the wall? Sure you have. And every time you thought, "Damn, I need some of those." Jennifer's whole life has been one big laminated plaque. She grew up in a house on whose walls hung her father's and her grandfather's awards, dated men whose walls hung heavy as well, and finally got up the courage to go after a mahogany plaque or two herself. Stop by and use her guest bathroom sometime and you will be quite dazzled by her accomplishments. They line the walls of that small room.

So, is it hard to get plaqued? Not at all. Often it is simply a matter of positioning yourself as the person who should be awarded something. Why would you want an award or an honor? Because they can look pretty cool on a résumé, on your office wall, or at some later point in your life, decorating your guest bathroom. Here are a few artful ways Jennifer has received awards, learned from the men in her life:

Enter the contest. Yes, simple as it is, try to win something. All too often women quite literally don't enter the contest of life. So if there is a professional competition that you daydream of winning, please don't delay. Enter the darn thing. Do you need to be nominated by someone else in order to be considered? Hard as it is, get over your shyness and ask that person to nominate you. Chances are he or she will be flattered and happy to help you.

Take credit. Don't be shy. If you want to be recognized, you will need to be able to claim your work as your own. Make sure everyone knows about your new innovative approach to an old problem, or your new product idea, or the way you landed that big sale.

Volunteer your time. Working for free can sometimes pay off in other ways. Volunteering in political campaigns is a great way to add to your career skills, meet interesting people, and gain useful connections. Many of Jennifer's big glossy plaques are thank-yous from various politicians, including a fancy framed letter from the White House for her help on a local project (not exactly a plaque, but still a big honor). She sometimes dated across party lines—one boyfriend was the president of the Berkeley College Republicans—and knowing people on both sides of the fence is always very useful.

Join the board. Raise your hand and say that you will serve. Yes, you will be the vice president of publicity; sure, you will be the sergeant at arms; and why not also head the new committee while you are at it? Serving on boards will get you noticed, and when your term is over, if you don't get a plaque, you will at least get a nice letter suitable for framing.

Invent an organization. Yes, this, too, is a great way to rise to the top, simply because you start out at the top. Create a club, start a cause, open a regional chapter of a national organization. This way you can appoint yourself the president and start adding ranks below. Make sure your organization has a great logo that will look nice engraved on an award.

Join a team. And maybe your team will win! Join a work team or a sports team and contribute as much as you can. See our lesson on How to Be a Team Player in chapter 7.

Give money. Crass, but true. Whenever you can afford to donate to a cause or a philanthropic organization you believe in, do so. Not only will you feel good about yourself and your contributions, but you also just might bring yourself to the attention of the sorts of people who will ask you to join boards, organize fund-raisers, and, hey, give out awards and plaques.

Stick around. Sometimes the best way to be honored is simply to stay around longer than anyone else.

PUT YOUR KNOWLEDGE TO **WORK**

Winning awards, being recognized by an organization, or being publicly thanked can be very useful ways to bring yourself up a rung or two on the career ladder. When starting out in a job, always join the professional organizations available to you, always volunteer to organize a new committee or serve on the board, and always show up at the meetings. And then when you start to collect awards and honors, always hang them prominently on your office walls where your boss can see them. Let your in-house newsletter editor know what you've won, and for good measure, send out a press release to the business section of your local paper. Work it for all it is worth.

How to Smoke a Cigar

Jennifer learned to smoke cigars from a diplomat. Can't you just picture it? A smoke-filled room populated by sober and well-educated men representing various governments and factions, puffing away at a leisurely pace while trying to settle their differences. Ah, does that ever happen anymore or has a scene like that slipped away for good?

Jennifer's personal diplomat, Jivan, is a cigar aficionado and is currently stationed in Vienna. Occasionally he even shows up in the pages of the magazine of the same name.

The best way to choose a good cigar is to throw yourself on the mercy of a cigar merchant. He will get a big thrill out of the opportunity to help a woman choose her first cigar (and he knows that if you enjoy it, you will come back over and over again). Spend some time; don't rush it.

If you don't like the way it smells in a cigar store, you will not like actually smoking a cigar. A taste for cigarettes (or a tolerance for cigarette smoke) doesn't have much bearing on whether you will enjoy the cigar-smoking ritual.

Cuban cigars are mostly delicious and give you a thrilling feeling of derring-do (because they are actually against the law in the United States), but there is nothing wrong with cigars from the Dominican Republic. Many of the growers came from Cuba anyway, with Cuban tobacco seed hidden in their pockets. Jivan started

CAUTION
Jennifer smokes Cubans when she can do it legally—outside U.S. borders, that is—but listen up, customs people, she does not try to bring them into the country and doesn't think anyone else should try, either. What seems like a sneaky and thrilling idea when you are packing to leave will end up a sweat-drenched and nervous way to get back into the country. Why risk having your vacation end badly when you get busted?

Jennifer on the Avo brand, and just the same way young girls stay with the same laundry soap their mother recommended, she only smokes Avos.

Few things are as calm and pleasurable as sitting next to your man in a cigar bar, smoking and talking. George Bingham and Jennifer have met several times for a cup of strong Cuban coffee and hand-rolled cigars in the same downtown Sacramento cigar bar that sends a courier to deliver a few to Governor Arnold every so often.

Okay, Jennifer will admit it: what she likes about cigar smoking (and the only thing she ever liked about cigarettes) are the accessories. She owns two vintage humidors, a graceful gold china cigar ashtray, and a cupboard of cognac snifters to go along with the moment. Get acquainted with a cigar shop and the little things they sell there and you will never be out of ideas for men's gifts.

Simple Steps to Smoking a Cigar

Cut off the end of the cigar—you can have the cigar-store guy do this for you. The unclipped part is what you will light; the newly clipped part is what you put to your lips.

Unlike a cigarette, a cigar takes a while to light. It's best to "warm" the tobacco by first passing a flame over the end and rotating it a bit to make sure all of the end has been warmed before you begin to puff on it. Put it between your lips and draw in, but don't puff. It might take a few matches to get the entire end burning, and you do need to make sure the entire end is lit, otherwise it will burn unevenly.

Cigars are not inhaled; you just puff on them and draw the smoke in and then exhale. Don't draw it all the way into your lungs or you will be doubled over, racked with a coughing fit. Once your cigar is nicely lit and you are puffing pleasantly away, try to keep the ash on the end, as that helps keep the smoke cool. Old cigar hands are the ones sitting with a big, long gravity-defying ash at the end of their cigars. "Nice ash," a stranger in a cigar bar once said to Jennifer, and she blushed with pride.

How to Get a Tattoo You Won't Regret

Although women have increasingly tatted their bodies over the last two decades, tattoos used to be reserved for sailors or servicemen. Shows like *LA Ink* display the nouveau emphasis on the female tattoo artist and the recipients of the tattoos. Regardless, tats are still a male-dominated art form with thousands of years of tribal roots. Lynne *never* considered getting a tattoo before meeting Stev Zachary. After all, her former husband, a force recon Marine turned operative, believed in "No identifying features!" But then she saw Stev's tattoos, which he had created himself, and was intrigued. For the first time, she saw a tattoo as a Michelangelo or a Botticelli—instead of some sagging rose on a former biker chick's breast or the name in a heart on the forearm of a man who had long since left his lover. As her friendship with Stev grew, she actually developed an appreciation for why one might tattoo his or her body. And so she is thinking about it . . .

Before you consider a tattoo, follow these tips:

- Make sure your tattoo has meaning to you. It's great to get a tattoo to commemorate a dead friend, but it can also leave you sad whenever you see it. It's more about personal expression than anything. What means the most to you? Lynne knew a devout Greek Orthodox girl who had a Byzantine cross tattooed on her wrist. Stev's tattoos are his jersey number on his back (soccer is his passion) and designs on his sides and chest that he himself drew. They are his own creation, like a painting.

Never get initials or names of boyfriends on your body. Even if you think it's forever, it might not be. You don't want to explain the "Jake" on your bum to every guy you ever date after Jake took off with a stripper.

- Don't pick a tattoo off the wall of the tattoo shop. Chances are two hundred other people sport the same picture. No individuality comes from copying what's on the wall. Bring your art to the artist.

- Speaking of the tattoo artist, don't just let anyone tattoo you. Talk to people with tattoos that you like and ask who the artist is. In Stev's case, he found two completely random people over a few weeks in a mall and asked each where and who did their respective work. Both people had the same tattoo artist.

- Talk to the tattoo artist. Again, Stev not only spoke with the artist recommended by the strangers but also sought out several artists in different shops. The one he chose took the time to speak with him for three hours about the process, healing, and his choice of tattoos, and he also showed Stev his work. "You've got to have a good rapport with the artist if you're going to trust him with a permanent work on your body," says Stev.

- Once you're comfortable with the artist, Stev recommends asking the artist if the tattoo you desire should include or omit anything. Get the artist's advice. You don't have to go with it, but a really talented artist will know when something isn't right or needs tweaking. If you've done your homework, you're in good shape and can feel confident about the work you're about to receive. "A really talented artist might want to change your idea a little and put his own twist to it," says Stev. "Let him if you feel comfortable and trusting. You'll end up with something that expresses who you are but better."

- Get ready for the pain. According to Stev, it's different for each person and depends upon the size of the implement used. Single needles hurt less, but take forever. In his case, the artist used a 44-needle device to fill in the tribal-like tattoos he drew. Even with the larger needle, each side took three hours, his chest took three hours, and his back took two hours. He explains the feeling as a "hot sting."

Your body is going to try to reject the ink. Be prepared to have seepage of color on your sheets and clothing for a while until your body accepts the ink.

- Once your tattoo is complete, the artist covers it in plastic wrap, and it's up to you to care for it.

PUT YOUR KNOWLEDGE TO WORK

Steve recommends A+D ointment for the healing process. The rate at which you heal is entirely dependent upon the size of the tattoo and your ability to heal. When you shower, use water only, no soap. Dab on the ointment and cover the tat with plastic wrap. Then cover your body with clothing. The less you scab, the better the result. Keep the tattoo moist with the ointment and covered until your skin heals.

7

Communications Studies

Women and men never seem to understand each other. This section helps bridge the gap and gives you great insight into how men communicate. Use the lessons to improve your career and your love life.

You hear it all the time—men and women speak a different language! In some ways, we do. Everything from nature vs. nurture to the hormones coursing through our bodies causes the difference in communication styles between the sexes. But just because girls are nurtured to speak less aggressively doesn't mean we cannot be team players or call a guy. In the School of Communications Studies you'll learn not only the vital differences between men and women but how to take your cue from men for more success in both the business world and your personal relationships.

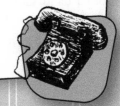

How to Talk about Yourself

Jennifer can tell you down to the smallest detail about the Southern California childhood of her former love George Bingham. He'd sit back in the faded velvet chairs in her living room and tell her about waves he'd surfed, Frisbees he'd tossed, and touchdowns he'd made on the high school football field. As the years went by she listened to a great many of those wistful memories. If pressed, she could recite a long list of his adult accomplishments, too, deals he'd closed and contracts he'd negotiated. Quite the powerful and accomplished businessman, that George.

Can he recite equally detailed stories about her Northern California girlhood? No. Can he list the high points of her publishing career? Nope, can't do that, either. It isn't his fault, though, because she didn't tell him. It simply never occurred to her that he'd be interested. Like many women, she worried that if she shared a story about herself that went on too long, his attention would drift and she'd find him fidgeting a bit in those overstuffed chairs, staring out the window wondering if maybe it was time to get back to the office.

Listening to George talk on and on about himself finally wore thin. However did he do it? She began to notice that George just talked and confidently assumed she'd be interested in whatever he was saying. Finally she plunged in and joined him. Maybe George doesn't know that much about her childhood, but everyone she dated after him does!

Women and men, girls and boys. We sit quietly and smile while they talk endlessly about themselves . . . on and on without ever stopping to wonder if anyone is really interested. Women, on the other hand, all too often assume that no one really wants to hear them talk about themselves. Does this hold us back when it comes to winning a promotion or being given a plum assignment? Yes, it does. So it is time to get over it, girls, and learn from the big boys just how it is done.

GO AHEAD, TALK ABOUT YOURSELF ALREADY

The first and most obvious thing Jennifer learned from all those one-sided conversations is that you just have to go ahead and start talking. Are you willing to try this method now? Here is an easy way to get started:

Head down to the grocery store and pick up an item or two.

As you stand in the checkout line, the clerk will say, "Howzit going?"

Jump right in and start talking; they are paid to be polite and listen.

Tell the grocery clerk exactly how your day was. If that doesn't take long, why not throw in a story from your childhood? "You know, this one time when I was ten I went to the store . . ."

A good trick is not to look at your audience that often, as it helps you focus on yourself and your story. You also won't notice that they are glancing down at their watches and are eyeing the exit. Remember, you are focusing on yourself, not on what you think they are thinking about you.

Is this selfish? You bet it is. Is it rude? It can be. It can also be a skill that you need to both acquire and refine in order to better maneuver through life.

TALK SOME MORE ABOUT YOURSELF

Ready for more lengthy periods of talking about yourself? First, put some time and effort into exactly what you want to say about yourself and how best to say it. Skip the never-ending story of what happened to you in the seventh grade with your former best friend and how she . . . oh never mind, even we're not interested in that one. If this is a business situation, choose a story that will cast you in a positive light and make you look like a leader, a creative thinker, and a determined problem solver. Something about a problem that you had to fix on your own, maybe? A flat tire on a deserted road, or the time you had to rescue your younger brother from impending disaster?

If you are too hesitant to start in on yourself right away, go ahead and soften up your audience by asking about them. "Tell me a story from when you were a little boy" is one of Jennifer's reliable ways to soften a man's heart (is it any wonder she knows so much about their childhoods, then?). Limit their time, though. Give them a few minutes to warm up before you swerve in with an anecdote of your own and steer the focus back to *you.*

Just plunge ahead and keep talking. Vanquish all thoughts of inadequacy and fear of bragging. Men do it all the time and it doesn't seem to be holding them back much, does it?

How to Feign Interest in a Much Younger Date

Yes, you might find yourself in this situation someday, so why not pick up a few clues from men who manage to sit quite happily gazing into the eyes of a date who is much, much younger than they are? Sure, the smooth young skin is a payoff later in the evening, but in the meantime, what the heck are you going to talk about?

As we mentioned earlier, one of Jennifer's ex-boyfriends was a teensy bit younger than she was. Just a tad. On the other hand, one of her former loves was so much older than she was that she never did bother to ask him exactly how old he was because she was afraid of what the answer might be . . . twenty years older? Thirty? Her age didn't seem to stop him from being terribly interested and seemingly entranced by all she had to say. Was he really listening? Who knows? Lynne recently dated a man fifteen years younger, and she proudly told him her age, offering it like a fine wine for him to enjoy.

"The Beatles? Honey, there used to be four of them . . ." Jennifer once overheard an exasperated gray-haired man tell his much younger date in a wine bar. We hope the conversation soon turned from music to recently released movies, or neither of them would have gotten much from the conversation they were working hard to have. The best conversations with a new acquaintance can involve discovering mutual interests and knowledge, the fact that you both went to camp in the eighth grade, and that you both had mono, too. But if one of you has been in the eighth grade more recently than the other, it can get awkward if actual dates and times come up in the conversation.

There are two different approaches to this situation:

1. Ask him about himself and let him talk while you add comments where you can. Try to stay away from observations that begin, "When I was your age . . ." Instead just keep asking him to extend his anecdotes by saying, "Wow. And then what happened?" "Were you grounded long when your parents found out?" or "Did the SAT people ever let you take the test again?" Lynne started her conversation off with, "Let's play twenty questions!" That way she seemed interested as she came up with questions about her new friend's life.

2. Just spend the whole night talking about yourself, your life, and your interests while not dwelling on whether it might not only bore him but also make you seem ancient when you

mention a band you loved in high school or which president you voted for two terms ago. If you use this method, you must feel entirely confident that one of the major reasons this very young person has decided to go out with you is that he is dazzled by your mature sophistication and awed by your many career accomplishments.

How to Understand Obscure Literary References

You know this man, too, don't you? The one who looks out at the quiet lake scene before you and sighs loudly and says, "So very, very Thoreau." Maybe you caught the reference to Henry David Thoreau and his book *On Walden Pond*, or maybe you didn't. You can't know everything. Lynne and Jennifer are no strangers to books; they have logged many a late-night hour with a classic novel. They have also logged a lot of time with literary men and secretly made notes on the offhand and knowing references that came up in conversation so you can get them, too.

As an obscure literary aside (see, we can do it, too), since everyone, even George W. Bush, claims to have read Albert Camus's *The Stranger*, should you ever hear anyone mention she's had a Camusian day, you'll know she's referring to existentialism, the philosophy inherent to the novel.

Why do you need to know these things? In just one summer morning reading the *Wall Street Journal* you would have had to understand the references to Manichaean (in an article about Harry Potter) and Aristotelian (the writer was talking about a bourbon).

Here are the cheat notes to help you with that:

Shavian refers to anything having to do with the English playwright George Bernard Shaw. He wrote *Pygmalion,* which was later the basis for the musical *My Fair Lady.*

Brobdingnagian is from Jonathan Swift's *Gulliver's Travels* and refers to anything of extraordinary size. In the book, the country of Brobdingnag was a country of giants.

Dickensian is derived from Charles Dickens. If a factory is referred to as Dickensian, it is because it is dark and crowded and dirty and lots of small children work there. But if some guy makes a Dickensian reference to you as a Miss Havisham, slug him and run.

Aristotelian is related to the Greek thinker and teacher Aristotle. An "Aristotelian mean" is a proper balance between things.

Manichaean (or Manichean) means to see the world in terms of good and evil, without any shading in between.

Hemingwayesque refers to, yes, Ernest himself. The term usually describes terse or spare language, or some sort of manly action. Fishing, hunting, waving a red flag in front of a bull, that sort of thing.

PUT YOUR KNOWLEDGE TO WORK

At the office you can easily work in references to Machiavellian or Manichaean behavior. Or why not work a reference to Aristotle into the next problem-solving meeting—"Can't we reach a more Aristotelian solution to this situation"—and leave everyone wondering where you did your semester abroad.

Machiavellian derives from the author of a book called *The Prince*, an Italian politician philosopher named Niccolò Machiavelli. It refers to any sort of behind-the-scenes maneuvering for control.

Jamesian would probably be Henry James, not his brother William. It could be about Americans naively making their way in Europe, or about social codes and standards.

Danteesque usually refers to Dante's description of hell and the circles surrounding it, or perhaps to his great devotion to his love, Beatrice. The first ring of hell, by the way, is for lovers—fornicators. They are whipped around, unable to touch each other for eternity. Pleasant, eh?

Whitmanesque is a reference to Walt Whitman. Poetry, don't you know, *Leaves of Grass* and so forth. He wrote during America's Romantic era of literature when nature was considered good and pure. Whitman's writings are primarily a reaction to industrialism.

Feel like showing off or trying to confuse or perhaps even intimidate? Go ahead and make up your own term; just add "esque" or "ish" or "ian" to the end of whichever writer you are alluding to.

Extra Credit

Watch reruns of *Frasier* and write down the references you don't get. Look them up online for an instant literary finishing course. It's also a great way to pick up wine and opera knowledge. Frasier and Niles can be your make-believe sophisticated boyfriends who bestow all of this upper-crust knowledge. These would be Crane-ian references, so to speak.

How to Be a Team Player

Be a team player! Join the team and add your strengths! Everywhere you turn in the corporate world nowadays someone is yammering on about team building. Which is all very well and good, unless you have never actually been on a team. What if the sport you excelled at was more solitary, like, say, knitting?

Jennifer is, um, not a team player. Sporty to be sure, but not in a teamlike manner. She runs alone in the woods every morning; her only teammates are coyotes and quail. So whenever she is urged to be a "team player," she falls back on the advice of her high school boyfriend Chris Cable, who was a talented tennis player. He was such a good team player that he and his doubles partner became the state champions.

"Team sports was a big teaching tool about life when I was growing up. I learned about cooperation, fair play, sportsmanship, and dealing with other people," Chris says now. Well, good for him. What about the rest of us, who hung out on the gym bleachers and hoped the teacher wouldn't notice we weren't playing?

Don't worry, Chris will explain it all for us.

First, it is important that you have something to offer to the rest of the team. You need to bring a skill or a talent that will strengthen the team as a whole. Try to figure out where you can best add to the folks who are already on the team and stress your abilities.

Second, you need to have an interest or a passion for

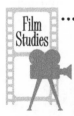
Film Studies

Okay, want to learn how to be more of a team player? Sit on the couch with your boyfriend and watch the remake of *The Longest Yard*. Or find the original version with Burt Reynolds. Younger crowds might enjoy the British version with Jason Statham, titled *Mean Machine*. Instead of football, the sport is what we Americans call soccer.

what the group is doing. If you don't, you add nothing. There is no point in being a part of a team whose mission doesn't move you.

Third, be a good listener. But also understand that you will need to speak up at times. You will need to feel comfortable brainstorming and taking the chance that some of your ideas might strike others as kind of weird. Keep going. Think out loud and encourage everyone else to do the same.

And last, follow through. As a team member it is critical that you do your part in the greater mission. Recognize when someone passes you the ball. On a playing field you will know when this happens: the ball is headed your way. In a business setting, it might be far more subtle, so watch for it.

If you have a team, someone needs to be in charge of it. Why not you? Step right up and let everyone else know that you want to lead the way. Without a leader, without established rules, a team will not accomplish anything other than a lot of wasted meetings.

And if you are the one building the team, make sure that the team actually has some authority. In a business setting, as well as in a sport setting, team members need to know that they exist for a reason. They need to know that they will be heard and that the work they do counts. Otherwise it will be a demoralizing waste of time, sort of like much of what seems to go on at the office . . .

PUT YOUR KNOWLEDGE TO WORK

Team building is not the time for you to fill the ranks with a lot of people you think are weak in the hope that it will make your own talents stand out. Wrong attitude. You want to stuff the ranks with people who are strong and talented so that your team will win and you will all shine. Got that? "I always made sure to play with people who were better than I was," Chris says. "How do you think I won the state championship?"

How to Use the NATO Phonetic Alphabet

Captain Jake Maloney flew fighters for the United States Navy and was truly a graduate of Top Gun. He met Lynne when she worked for a military insurer, USAA, during college. Although her father is a military pilot, she'd never learned about anything related to aviation until she met Jake, a friend of a friend who was suddenly stranded in Lynne's town and called her for help. She needed a way to instantly impress him with her knowledge. She'd long since learned that every pilot's first line out of the pickup gate is: "I'm a pilot." They all say it with confidence, as if it's supposed to magically make one swoon! Lynne's snotty response was always: "So what? My father's a Medevac pilot who flew in Vietnam. Try again." But something about this captain made her melt. She knew his "stranded" line screamed "Cheesy!" But she still gained permission from the master warrant officer, her dad, to settle him in the guest room for the night.

So how to impress him? In this case, she didn't let him teach her anything. In order to work for USAA, she'd needed to pass a NATO phonetic alphabet test, required to read back all letters to their clients using the phonetic alphabet. So Lynne gave him directions to her house, including her address, using the phonetic alphabet. What she didn't spell out for him until he arrived was this: "India. Lima, India, Victor, Echo. Alpha, Tango. Hotel, Oscar, Mike, Echo." *I live at home.* And then she introduced him to her dad!

WHAT IS THE NATO PHONETIC ALPHABET?

You know when you see a movie and the pilot uses strange words to spell out something? He's using the international radiotelephony spelling alphabet, more commonly referred to as the NATO phonetic alphabet. The phonetic alphabet is really a spelling alphabet. When one communicates by voice over a phone or a radio, sometimes interference causes a mishearing. With the prolific use of cell phones in our lives, we all know how difficult it often is to hear clearly. Not hearing the correct information in the military can prove deadly on a mission, during an emergency landing, or in an evacuation. Even in non-life-threatening circumstances, obtaining the correct information can help everyone avoid hassles.

HOW DOES IT WORK?

It's elementary, really. The NATO phonetic alphabet assigns code words to the letters of the English alphabet. No matter what the native languages of the people transmitting and receiving the critical message, the letters (and numbers) are pronounced correctly and understood because it's a uniform code. Typically, only critical parts of a message are spelled out using the NATO phonetic alphabet.

Let's say a tower needs to transmit that a plane is in the direct path of another plane. The plane in the direct path is a DC-10. In order to be perfectly clear, the air traffic controller might say, "Delta Charlie One Zero in twelve o'clock position." Whenever there's any doubt of the model of the aircraft, like a UH-I helicopter, for example (especially when the model is difficult to pronounce and doesn't always sound clear across the radio as is the case with the UH-I), the pilot and/or approach tower might specify "Uniform Hotel One."

The tail number of civil aircraft also has anywhere from one to three letters as identification. Let's say the aircraft's identification is 134RJ. The pilot calls the tower and announces his approach by identifying his craft as "One Three Four Romeo Juliet."

The most common use among pilots is probably the airport code. All airports around the world possess a unique, three-letter identifier. Orlando, Florida, for example, is MCO. The pilot will call out to "Mike Charlie Oscar" when contacting the tower.

HOW DID IT BEGIN?

In 1927, the International Telecommunication Union created the first phonetic alphabet. World War II brought about a similar phonetic alphabet used by Allied Forces called the Joint Army/Navy Phonetic Alphabet. Civilian aviation adopted its usage. Neither of these phonetic alphabets is used today because of problems found with the universality of the pronunciations. In 1956, however, after much testing, the International Civil Aviation Organization adopted what most organizations and military installations use. The name—NATO phonetic alphabet—first appeared in an Allied Tactical Publication, which was used by

PUT YOUR KNOWLEDGE TO WORK

While working in a small arts office as an accountant, a good friend and her colleagues overheard another employee in his cubicle speaking on the phone with the city about a grant check. The city official needed the employee to repeat back a series of numbers and letters on the paperwork for the check. Not knowing the universally recognized NATO phonetic alphabet, this male employee sent the otherwise all-female office into a fit of giggles when he said, "A, B, S, C, 1, 5, 3, 7. Yes, Aqua Boy Snorts Cats, One, Five, Three, Seven." Clearly, he used an original phonetic alphabet not recognized by the ICAO or NATO.

Let your office know you mean serious business and learn the NATO phonetic alphabet. Alpha, Bravo, Sierra, Charlie sounds so much more professional than Aqua Boy Snorts Cats—and it won't get the American Society for the Prevention of Cruelty to Animals knocking on the door, either.

all allied navies in NATO (North Atlantic Treaty Organization).

Because pronunciations vary by the language of the speakers, the International Civil Aviation Organization provides posters that illustrate proper pronunciation of all telephonics.

What follows is the NATO phonetic alphabet. Use it with pride to better communicate with everyone from your cell phone billing representative to your boss.

A—Alpha	U—Uniform	3—Three
B—Bravo	V—Victor	4—Four
C—Charlie	W—Whiskey	5—Five
D—Delta	X—X-ray	6—Six
E—Echo	Y—Yankee	7—Seven
F—Foxtrot	Z—Zulu	8—Eight
G—Golf	1—One	9—Niner
H—Hotel	2—Two	0—Zero
I—India		
J—Juliet		
K—Kilo		
L—Lima		
M—Mike		
N—November		
O—Oscar		
P—Papa		
Q—Quebec		
R—Romeo		
S—Sierra		
T—Tango		

Want to impress a guy in the military with your understanding of the nuances of the NATO phonetic alphabet? Many abbreviations of the code mean something different than what you'd expect. "Bravo Zulu" or even "BZ" stands for "Well done," and "Sierra Hotel" stands for "Shit hot," which is used widely by military men for "You're good!" If your guy does something that impresses you, tell him, "BZ, honey!" or if you can take the language and don't mind a little dirty talk, tell him you think he looks "Sierra Hotel."

PUT YOUR KNOWLEDGE TO W*o*RK

In your career, you might travel or desire to travel. Perhaps you deal with companies in different countries in many time zones. Especially if you're in a job within the governmental sector, your chances are good you'll have a boss with a military background. Impress him or her with your knowledge of both the NATO phonetic alphabet and time zones. Here's the lowdown you'll need:

- There are twenty-six time zones around the world, labeled A to Z.
- Greenwich Mean Time is in the "Z" zone.
- Greenwich Mean Time is referred to as merely "Zulu."
- The Prime Meridian just happens to run through this zone, so it's pretty popular—and just south of London, too.

So let's put it to use. Your boss is leaving on a trip to London, and you're in charge of the agenda. Tell him, "You'll be arriving at 13:45 Zulu." Translation: "You'll be arriving at 1:45 p.m., Greenwich Mean Time."

How to Get to the Point

Women. We are so great, don't you think? Maybe not in all ways, but in some ways, or at least most ways, depending on who is doing the thinking, perhaps. On the other hand, we all do spend so much time thinking about what to say, when to say what we want to say, how someone might react to what we have to say, whether they might be hurt by what we might want to say to them, and what on earth we will say when they say something back to us, and . . . sometimes it takes awhile for us to get the point, doesn't it? To come right out and say what is on our minds.

Lynne and Jennifer both dated direct, to-the-point, no-nonsense men. Jennifer married one. Lynne divorced one.

Envious of how the guys always seem to be able to just put

whatever they want to say out there and to hell with what any-one else thinks? That is a handy skill to have. So here, the next time you feel the need to speak up and say something to someone, try it this way: Something on your mind? Open your mouth and say it. Boom. It's over. Done. Say what you want to say and move on. Got it? Good. Cause we're done here.

How to Talk about Yourself Again

What? Already? Sure. You got away with it once; why not keep on doing it? What we have learned from a boyfriend or two is that being able to talk with confidence about yourself is an important element in professional success. If you can't talk about yourself and your accomplishments, you can't let an interviewer see that you are the perfect person for a job. In many ways, your future can rest on whether you have the confidence and courage to talk about your-self and your accomplishments when called upon to do it.

Humorist Fran Lebowitz once described a conversation as talk-ing and waiting for your turn to talk. So when it is your turn to talk, honey, go right ahead and don't yield the floor. And as for worrying if anyone is interested, or if anyone is listening, don't. Never, ever say: "Oh, I'm sorry. I've gone on about myself too long." No you haven't; you are just warming up!

If you need to ease into this habit, why not schedule a practice session with your girlfriends? Put a timer in the middle of the table and let everyone have an uninterrupted five minutes of "me" time.

Jennifer is a huge fan of the speaking club Toastmasters International. Participating in weekly meetings gives you a chance to practice talking about anything, including yourself. In fact, the very first speech that all members must give is called the icebreaker, in which you talk about yourself and introduce yourself to the club members. Check it out; there are clubs all over the world, and your confidence will soar once you perfect your public speaking skills. Their Web site is www.toastmasters.org.

Write a two-paragraph description of your best-ever accomplishment at work. See how you can shape it into a story that will cast you and your skills in a good light. Practice it on your dog, your mother, your letter carrier. And then give it a try at work.

What makes a good story is this: a bit of a setback, followed by an eventual (and hard-won) triumph. Make sure that you don't appear to be superhuman in the way you portray yourself; show a few warts (metaphorically speaking, of course!). It will endear you to your listener.

The next time you're at a gathering of your colleagues, listen closely for an opening. You could tag your comment onto a current event or a recent headline, a trick every publicist knows. "The trouble in the Middle East reminds me of the time I . . ." and then launch into a story about wonderful you.

How and When to Call Men

Max Constantine was a boyfriend of few words. Unless Lynne was with him, she wasn't necessarily speaking to him. You wouldn't find Max on the phone, murmuring sweet nothings, *ever*. His calls to Lynne were infrequent and concise, as were his text messages, which were reserved for occasional sexy notes. Lynne, however, speaks, talks, and loves her unlimited minutes and texting feature. A consummate storyteller, Lynne couldn't quite adjust to this man of few words. In his eyes, she seemed like Glenn Close's character in *Fatal Attraction*. In Lynne's eyes, Max appeared removed, unfeeling, insensitive, closed. Neither description rings true for either. Interestingly, Max has been the only guy in Lynne's life to recognize her true feelings and see through her strong personality to get to her more fragile aspect. And *twice* (granted, over the span of a few months), Lynne called him, declaring (half jokingly, half truthfully), "You don't love me anymore!" when her calls or texts weren't immediately returned by Max. The first time, he called assuaging her fears, "Of course I love you. I'm just a jerk who never talks on the phone." The second time? We'll leave that for the lesson!

Technology! What a convenience! We stay in contact with so many people so quickly. Everyone is now a mere e-mail, text message, or cell phone call away, accessible wherever they stand on the globe at any moment. Unfortunately, the interaction of men and women because of all this technology has become more complicated. It's no longer a simple message left on a home answering machine when your lover isn't at home.

Because technology makes communication so convenient, phone calls don't seem as weighted as they did in the past, either. Ask any teen or twentysomething—texting especially is de rigueur.

Extra Credit

Now, if you really want to take a male approach to this whole phone/text thing, decide to become a player. Text and phone as many guys as you want, frequently. Throw out all the love you can and catch what comes back. Remember, do this only if you really don't care too much about any of the guys (if you care at all!). That way, it won't be disappointing if no one returns your silly messages or texts. In fact, receiving a barrage of male attention isn't the worst thing for one's ego. Lynne, not currently aligning herself with any one particular boyfriend, especially likes to text her beaux or leave breathy voice mail messages. Invariably, she'll receive several ego boosts from her few minutes of effort. So go ahead if you're impervious to feeling anything for any of the guys. We highly recommend "playing" phone and text tag.

Two people don't necessarily share romantic ideations to text each other ten times in one day. Communication remains far more fluid with this set.

We both learned one generation of boyfriends' lessons regarding when to phone years ago and needed to go back to night school in the twenty-first century to get more Boyfriend University credits regarding phone and text etiquette. That's why we've compiled the knowledge learned from several guy friends, not just Max.

Follow these rules so as not to cause your man to throw his phone in the lake just to avoid you:

- You can call him *if* he gives you his number and tells you to call.

- Don't worry about waiting an obligatory number of days. Call when it feels comfortable to you. If he answers and sounds happy to hear from you, you're in. Most men admit to letting the phone go to voice mail if they're not interested.

- You can also wait for him to call you (assuming you've given him your number).

- Send a short text message if you aren't ready to call. If you receive a response within twenty-four hours, it's cool to text again.

- If he doesn't return your first text with either a phone call or another text, walk away and decide not to waste your emotions or time on this guy.

- If he calls you first, great! You know he likes you and you can begin to judiciously call or text him—every few days at first, as long as he's responding.

- After your first few interactions, if you want to know how serious he is, don't call or text him until he calls or texts you.

Give yourself a time frame in which he must call for it to be acceptable for you to call him back or answer. Lynne's friend Marianna allows a three-day window. If he hasn't called within three days, she lets it—and him—go.

- But what if he calls after the three-day time line? Marianna says, "Then I don't answer him immediately. I let him leave three messages before I return the call." Strong girl. Most guys we spoke with regarding this measure smiled, acknowledging that the chase meant something, but they made it clear that they wouldn't call three times.

- If you're only texting because you believe you'll vomit from fright by calling, this isn't a relationship you can pursue. Don't even text. You need to get comfortable in your own skin before you can roll the emotional dice of phone play.

- Don't assume that just because he hasn't called in a day or two he doesn't adore you. Remember Max? Lynne's second "You don't love me!" speech came when she hadn't heard from him in a few hours short of a day! Max just laughed and called, telling Lynne, "Of course I still love and adore you. Not everyone keeps his phone attached to him all day. Some of us only check our messages once a day, believe it or not!" You'll know within a few weeks of the relationship if he's a talker, a texter, or neither.

- Regardless, if you really like the guy, don't inundate him with calls or texts—*ever*. One call a day at most. Two or three texts a day is max for the younger crowd, which sustains itself on constant texting. Older guys don't want all the texts or calls.

- If you haven't heard from him in a few days, don't text the guy incessantly. If you do, call a friend to stop you! Round up a support group you can depend on to tell you, "Walk away from the phone. Step away from the text."

- If you do bombard the man with phone or text messages, regain your dignity and lie low. Don't call. Don't text. Let him call or text you. He will if he likes you.

- If the whole phone/text thing is still killing you, it's time to get direct. Call and ask, "What are we doing? What is this?" Yep, time to define the relationship or you'll condemn your-self to texting purgatory for way too many months, wasting money and time on the bum who might be playing you the way Lynne plays men.

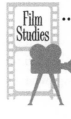

Film Studies

Luckily, ladies, men aren't immune to the phone/text panic. When a guy truly likes you, nothing stops him from calling. In fact, we bet that if you don't like the guy, he'll call and text you incessantly. Nevertheless, take your cue from the following lines from *Swingers*, starring Vince Vaughn and Jon Favreau, if you really want a look at the male perspective:

"How about if I wait six weeks to call. I could tell her I found her num-ber while I was cleaning out my wallet, I can't remember where we met. I'll ask her what she looks like and then I'll ask her if we f——. How about that? Would that be money?"

How to Cry Like a Guy: The Crying Game

"Tears, idle tears, I know not what they mean," wrote Alfred, Lord Tennyson. Lynne learned what they mean to men after a small altercation between a best friend and her beau at the time, Mark Potter. Mark, Lynne learned, held strong feelings about women crying. Unfortunately, Lynne's friend Barbara was on a crying jag over a divorce when Mark brought up his belief that "women use crying as manipulation." He saw crying as any female's way to get the guy to soften during a fight. A strong-willed woman, Barbara blasted Mark with her own feelings on the subject, telling Mark, "It's not always about you. We aren't necessarily crying in front of anyone in order to manipulate them." Weeks later, Barbara confided to Lynne that she "hated" Mark. Lynne never exposed Barbara to Mark. Mark called Barbara smug, believing he just told her what she didn't want to hear. In reality, both Barbara and Mark are right. The real answer lies somewhere in the middle.

Lynne's not one of those women to cry over just anything. She typically reserves her tears for death and trauma to her children. That's it. Barbara, however, cries about more things. Another coworker of Lynne's claims to cry at Campbell's soup commercials if she's about ready to start her period. Consequently, we cannot have the "crying game" conversation without first raising two fundamental differences between men and women:

1. **Nature vs. nurture.** Nature gives us all the ability to cry, but add female hormones (over which we have limited control) and society's nurturing of males *not* to cry and you've achieved a weighty difference between the sexes. From boyhood, young men are told to "buck up" and "walk it off." They're not really allowed to cry after a particularly rough game or day. Girls, however, can cry. No one stops us necessarily. Men are considered weak if they cry. Women? Not so much—unless they're dating Mark!

2. **Chemical release.** Did you know that we all release serotonin when we cry, which actually helps make us happier? Yep, our bodies release the exact chemical that chemists have tried to duplicate in Prozac!

With that off the table, let's look at the male perspective regarding crying and a few rules you might want to follow:

- Lynne talked to several men, who all confirmed that men only cry at some deaths and the death of their dog. Only death remains an acceptable time for most men to cry.

- Does this mean that men believe that women should only cry at death and that anything else is manipulation? No. But men are less tolerant of crying than you might believe. For those familiar with the hit comedy *Seinfeld*, you might remember a famous episode where Jerry is floored by a girl who will cry at her shoelace's breaking or a problem with her food but brushes off the death of a family member. The other tears seem "idle" (thank you very much, Lord Tennyson), whereas at what would appear a perfectly acceptable time to cry—death—the girl remains unmoved.

- Never use crying as manipulation, but never let a guy dictate when you do or don't cry. If he doesn't like your crying after *ER*, tell him to go in the other room. If you're more like Lynne and can't cry, kudos! Only you decide when to cry, baby.

- Never judge a man if he doesn't cry—or come immediately to comfort you when you do. Men aren't nurtured to cry or understand the cry response. He doesn't necessarily know that you want him to cradle you in his arms for a whopper waterworks! If you need holding, tell him. He cannot read your mind. Most men don't mind giving a little love once in a while to a crying girlfriend or wife.

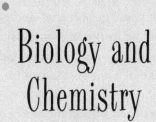

8

Biology and Chemistry

Ah! The differences between the sexes. You want to know the man's perspective regarding things sexual. Look no further.

Lynne's parents met in high school chemistry class. We guess the chemistry between the two worked! Navigating the differences biologically and chemically between men and woman can prove daunting today. We live in a world of the "noncommitted committed" relationship. "What?" you might ask. Well, we've been pulled through the sexual and feminist revolution with a now-aggressive impact of Internet pornography and the advent of Viagra. Not to mention, though he looks more like the Crypt Keeper these days, Hugh Hefner has three girlfriends. Honestly, understanding sex, pleasure, attraction, love vs. lust vs. longing, and more isn't necessarily clear to either men or women.

Consequently, more and more women we know exist in these relationships where they don't know just how committed they are to the men or the men to them. What we came to understand in our collective dating lives is to live by this motto: I came, I dated, I conquered. To win at this love game, you might need to readjust your "girl-ometer" and go for the guy approach. If you learn how he works relationships, you'll not only intrigue your man ("She doesn't do the typical girl things? I don't understand it but I like it!") but also learn a ton about making yourself content sexually.

Come on! Sex is an important aspect of our survival. Just ask Maslow; it's right up there with food and shelter. This section provides useful advice on everything from flaunting your assets to accepting pleasure. Get comfortable between the sheets, because we plan to teach you a few tricks!

How to Hide Bad Behavior

We have both gone out with men adept at hiding everything from their infidelity to their drinking to more. Unfortunately, this lesson isn't taught so much by the guys' actually possessing an interest in giving you the knowledge. You just wise up and see a pattern, as Jennifer did with a guy who would always manipulate his excuses to make it appear as if Jennifer was the person who got the information wrong. Or you ask a good, truthful male, as Lynne did, about what the XY-chromosomal type does to hide his terrible vices.

THE EXCUSER

Learn how to make excuses that are ambiguous, and at the same time turn them toward the person to whom you are offering an excuse. Here are the two key phrases to use:

1. I didn't get your message.
2. Oh, I didn't know we had firmed up any plans.

The "I didn't get your message/e-mail/text" excuse makes it appear as if you would have responded or been interested, at any rate, had you only received it! "Oh, I didn't know we had firmed up any plans" makes it sound as if your not materializing at a party/event/home was truly merely a miscommunication. How can one possibly get angry at the absence if the "excuser" didn't have a clue that he was supposed to be there? One of Jennifer's boyfriends used this excuse for a family-planned holiday dinner. Sure, he was a creep who was actually with another girl at the time, but he hid that bad behavior. If you plan on ignoring a message or an invitation, turnabout is fair play. Learn from the guys, girls.

THE CHEATER

These techniques were developed, used, and divulged by a good friend of Lynne's who shall remain nameless to protect his identity from other dudes. Use them to keep any extracurricular "activities" from your boyfriend:

1. Guys' night out is often a way to get away from the girlfriend and enjoy the attention of other women—even if it doesn't lead to sex or a long-term affair. So ladies, enjoy lots of girls' nights out if you plan to cheat. "Hey, I'm having dinner with my girlfriends."

2. Turn your cell phone to silent if you're with another person. If you're in a public place, excuse yourself to use the restroom and call your boyfriend back. Tell him, "It was loud and I didn't hear the phone, but the second I saw I'd missed your call, I had to call you back, baby."

3. In your cell phone's address book, change the name of the guy you're cheating with to a woman's name. If it's "John," for example, list the name on your cell phone as "Joanie." If

John calls while you're with your boyfriend, say "I don't want to take her call. She's just some girl at work who wants to hang out." Now here's where it gets tricky. If John knows that you've got a boyfriend, no worries about changing your boyfriend's name on your phone when you're with John. If your boyfriend's name pops up, John won't care. Otherwise, you'll need to have fake names that you change back and forth between hooking up with each guy.

4. Always be where you're going to be when you say you're going to be there. If you're supposed to meet him at the restaurant at 7 p.m., for example, be there at 7 p.m. Lynne has a friend, Libby, who dated a cheater, but she never found out until much after the relationship because he was always on time for their dates, picked her up at work when he said he would, and never deviated from their plans. Whenever she had the slightest inkling he was cheating, he asked, with assurance, "Baby, am I always here when I say I'll be here?" or "Have I ever not been somewhere when I said I would?" This leads to the next concept . . .

5. Cheat while your man is at work or away altogether. Cheat on his time, not on yours. It's time for extracurricular activities when you know he's otherwise occupied.

6. Always cheat out of town, and never, ever give your "friend" your home address or go to his house. You don't want anyone unexpectedly arriving while you're visiting each other.

7 Avoid public places. One guy got caught at a Wendy's because the girl he was cheating with worked there and his girlfriend went to eat there with his mother. You never know how paths will cross or who will see you. Stay out of populated places.

8. Finally, take a shower after your rendezvous is over. Really. Don't have another man's scent on you.

When you are the one with the cheater, never try to teach him new tricks. One man known by one of us kissed horribly. But she didn't dare show him how she liked to be kissed because she knew ultimately he'd use it on his wife. Their liaison might suffer because the wife would pick up on the new technique. If you don't want to get caught, don't teach the old dog new tricks!

The best advice Lynne's friend gave her about hiding bad behavior was this: don't do anything you'll regret; know yourself. Nevertheless, if you want to lead the "bad girl" lifestyle, now you know how.

How to Accept Pleasure

This topic is a tough one for us. Yet the answer and the lesson are pretty simple—just not as easy to actually enact. We're talking about letting go sexually and allowing yourself sexual pleasure with no guilt, no inhibitions, and believing you deserve pleasure. Since this topic contains intimate information, Lynne and Jennifer won't tell you the tales of the moments in bed when they each respectively learned how to accept pleasure. Instead, here is information that'll help you enjoy your body like a man enjoys his, with some thoughts directly from a guy source or two:

- "Men take pleasure as a given, kind of like a dog sleeping in the sunlight. The sun is there. It feels good. The dog enjoys sleeping in the sun. Start thinking that pleasure is a given." When the opportunity arises, make use of it, ladies. Choose to enjoy the sun.

- "Men take pleasure like they expect it to be there." You need to decide that you will take pleasure. And you should definitely expect it to be there.

- "Let go of any inhibitions about your body. Men aren't thinking about anything during sex but the sex and enjoying it. Men don't worry about whether or not their ass is waxed and let that stop the flow of an orgasm." What this man just told us is to not worry about our bodies. If he's there with you, he's enjoying it and your body. And you need to enjoy it and his body.

- At the same time, focus on your body. Don't worry about anyone else's pleasure, nurturing, aid, or care. Because our bodies carry babies who maneuver through our vaginas to breathe life, we're mentally in tune with nurturing others through our sexual organs and arousal areas. Our breasts secrete milk for nourishment, for goodness' sake. One of the best lines in comedy was spoken by Murphy Brown when she realized that having her child would result in nursing. She exclaims in utter disbelief something like, "That's like telling me I'm going to have bacon come out of my elbow." Murphy held a decidedly more male approach to her body. Good for her. Nevertheless, our anatomy is designed for nurturing, giving—and sometimes we forget it's also designed for receiving.

- A male friend of Lynne's reasoned why he so easily accepts that he's going to be nurtured and pleasured: "I have no concept of what it's like to worry about somebody living in me but me. So I naturally assume that anything done to me or given to me is going to be a feel-good thing. I'm never 'outside' my own self." The dude may sound selfish, but do what he does: stay within your own body and *receive*.

- Once things start feeling good, just let go. Let go as you would on an amusement park ride. "I hope that any woman I'm with will feel so good that she just lets go to feel even more," said a former lover of Lynne's.

- Don't reject pleasure if it's offered. Never do something you feel morally uncomfortable with, but truly, have you ever known a man to move your hand away from his pants? Have you known many men to stop you when you begin arousing them? Don't stop the experience, ladies. He obviously wants to try to bring you pleasure; you won't ever know his talents if you stop him.

- "Go primal." Basically, what this guy told Lynne was to release yourself of all societal discomfort. Men "act a little bit more animal and it's okay." Men are taught to make jokes about bodily functions and accept them. Women are taught to hide everything. Because men don't have so many societal taboos, they can be a more natural and release a more primitive side that can be very sexy. Choose to go primal. Just a hint: you'll feel it in the way you look at your guy when it's happening.

Pleasuring yourself is an important aspect of "accepting pleasure like a man." How many stupid-guy flicks contain masturbation jokes? We don't think there's anything funny about masturbating. Instead, we think making sure you feel good remains instrumental to good health. Take your cue from the Divinyls tune "I Touch Myself," where the female lead singer openly lyricizes her pleasure needs and fixes.

Put simply, women have always taken care of everyone—physiologically speaking. We tend to focus on whether the man in our life receives the pleasure. That's okay. But it's not okay to relinquish your own pleasure. Take pleasure like a man!

When to Sleep with a Guy

When is it acceptable in a relationship to sleep with a guy? Well, that depends on what you want. You've probably already read the books that give you time lines of how many dates one must go on before engaging in sexual intercourse. One of Jennifer's friend's, Claudine, advises that she tells any guy she goes out with that her time line is six months! Yep, half a year before the prized encounter takes place. Claudine says, "It takes the pressure of sex off the table immediately." Without the pressure, she feels room to explore the person. Yet another friend of Lynne's, Rachel, sleeps with all her dates on the first date. "Please! It gets it out of the way. If he isn't a good lover, I don't want to waste my time with him!" says Rachel. This section provides a frank discussion of how men decide when to sleep with a woman and how you decide when the time is right.

A number can never provide the answer for everyone. Three dates? Six dates? First date? Six months? Have you ever met anyone who slept with her husband on the first date? We have. You might possess personal experience, however, on the opposite side of the equation. You really felt a connection with someone, threw

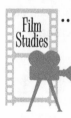

Film Studies

In the quote below, John Cusack's character in the film *High Fidelity* knows himself and speaks with wit and humor about sleeping with someone. He could've had sex and exorcised the rejection demons, but ultimately it didn't fit with his ways.

"I could've wound up having sex back there. And what better way to exorcise rejection demons than to screw the person who rejected you, right? But you wouldn't be sleeping with a person, you'd be sleeping with the whole sad, single-person culture. It'd be like sleeping with Talia Shire in *Rocky* if you weren't Rocky."

caution to the wind, and cuddled between the covers after mind-blowing sex. Now you're asking yourself, "Why doesn't he call?"

We hate to admit it, but we can't give you a simple answer here. There's no one answer. Perhaps, sadly, he's a player and used you. Perhaps he's madly in love with you and freaked out.

Nevertheless, how do you react to his not calling, and what can you live with? These are the questions you need to ask yourself when dealing with first encounters between the sheets.

THE CONQUEST

Let's get this out right now. Yes, most men like the chase. They want the conquest. Most men haven't left the anthropological phase of hunter. They hunt. They hunt women. But does that necessarily mean that once a guy "hits it" with you he hits the pavement and moves on to new prey? Absolutely not! In our lives, we've found the opposite to be true. Generally speaking, most men *do* call after a first date/sex date. Sure, there might have been a one-night stand or two within our lives, but here's where you act like the man. Buck up! Move on. If he doesn't call and you were just prey, consider what you got out of it. Did you orgasm? Did it feel good? Was it fun? Did you burn a few calories without having to hit the stupid gym? Find a reason to have gotten something out of the encounter instead of focusing on what you might have lost.

HOW SOON IS TOO SOON?

Neither of us held a hard line on the number of dates before we'd plunge into sex with a suitor. Some guys took longer than others. Here's the question: What can you live with? Because here's the reality: if you follow the six-month rule like Jennifer's friend Claudine, you might miss out on some sexually adventurous guy who'll also make you laugh and love him—but he leaves because he's not willing to wait six months for sex. On the other hand, if you're like Rachel, you might end up sleeping with many men who just desire one encounter. But if all you want is the knowledge of whether he floats your boat in bed, then sleeping with a guy on the first date is something you can live with. If, however, you desire more than a roll in the hay, this isn't the way to go. Thousands of lovesick women bemoan, "Why did I sleep with him so soon?" thinking they lost the love of their lives with this one act. *You didn't.* It may hurt, but lust isn't love, honey. Don't sell yourself short. He can never be the love of your life if he left you. Stop crying. Get up and find another guy.

The answer, then, to when should you sleep with a guy? Whenever you're comfortable and know that you'll be okay if he moves on after the sex.

We know. It is a tough question, because you need to know yourself and take joy in whatever experiences come your way. So figure out who you are and either give yourself a number or decide to act more fluidly and take sex on a case-by-case basis. It always feels best to do what you believe in . . . to follow your own credo about sex.

How to Avoid Getting Used in a Relationship

Lynne has a friend named Angela. They've been friends for twenty years, since high school. Unfortunately, most everything Lynne learned about not getting used in a relationship comes from watching Angela move men in and out of her life. Without describing all the men who've used this woman physically, emotionally, and financially (everyone from the thief to the gambler to the cheater and more), let's take a look at one. Angela has built a great career. She's successful in the business world. She also owns millions—yes, millions—in property. She's beautiful, funny, and talented. But when it comes to men, she just gets used. Recently, a guy in his forties with nothing but the clothes on his back moved himself into her waterfront property. Does he contribute? No. Is he necessarily good to her? Not unless you think controlling someone by estranging her from her best friends and constantly "borrowing" money for his jail stints and legal fees is being a good boyfriend. Really, dear reader, don't go too hard on Angela. We've all let men, even if briefly out of confusion between giving and taking, or through denial, use us. Though Angela secretly knows this guy isn't good, that he's using her, her denial and low self-esteem reach deep. In this section, we look at the user and how to avoid this guy. You're worth so much more than a man who doesn't respect you, your successes, or your finances. If you read this section and it reveals that you are indeed getting used by a guy, we

Extra Credit

Too often on radio talk shows, men call in claiming that women like to be treated like shit. A pal of Lynne's says that he's essentially disillusioned by most women. "Treat them well, and they treat you badly. Treat them terribly, and they come running."

The only way we women are going to stop getting used is by not allowing ourselves to be used. Banish the idea of the "bad boy" who mistreats you as hot and seductive. We're not talking about a guy with an edge (hot!—but only if he treats you with the same respect you show him). Real women—successful, empowered, beautiful women—don't allow men to play games with them, nor do they play games. Show a man your strength by expecting respect, and show him respect. If the guy you're seeing can't use you, he's either going to stop and appreciate the person you are or leave . . . and you don't want him anyway if that's the case.

urge you to look at it as an experiment. You observed like a scientist, collected the data. Now get out!

Let's begin with the basics. Men use women in many ways. The three biggies? (1) Physically, when he uses you for sex or just to impress his friends with your beauty or success but doesn't really enjoy you as a person, (2) financially, when there isn't equality concerning money, gifts, and so on, and (3) emotionally, when he doesn't reciprocate your emotions and the relationship is inauthentic. Here are the clues:

- If your "boyfriend" never introduces you to his friends or family, essentially doesn't integrate you into his life, you're being used. He might also be really uncomfortable about meeting your friends and family—another clear sign to get out.

- Be wary if there's a distinct, unvarying pattern to his availability. If he only calls you on certain days, and it's usually just for sex or money or whatever, he's probably in another relationship (or many others) and is using you. We highly recommend watching the FX series *Rescue Me* for insight into both the good and the bad ways men treat women.

- If he doesn't want you ever stopping by during a break at work, he's using you. If you're not allowed to just drop by his home, he's using you.

- If he plans major events, such as trips to the city, wineries in the country, professional sports games, or concerts, with his "buddies" but *never* with you, he's using you.

- Likewise, if he only brings you to social events and parades you around but never spends time with you alone, such as a quiet dinner at a restaurant, he's using you as a front. Perhaps he's receiving pressure from family to find a girl to settle down with or he's gay or you're amazingly beautiful and he wants his friends to think he's the alpha male (because they all know he's seeing other women, too!).

- If he's always asking you for things and never reciprocating, he's using you. "I asked a girl for a laptop for Christmas one year, because I knew she could afford it. I wasn't going to buy her much of anything," truthfully tells a "serial user." The girl bought the computer.

- If he bullies you into providing for his bills and his desires over your own, he's using you.

- If he only calls you back to ask if you want to come over and share a physical experience, he's using you.

- If he tells you that you have to leave the aforementioned liaison by a certain time and kicks you out of bed, he's using you.

- If he never brings you back to his place, and everything between you happens at your place, he's using you.

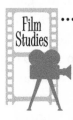

Film Studies

Want to receive easy, inexpensive lessons on the male psychology behind treatment of women? Look at characters in several "guy" movies or TV shows. Check out Tony Soprano in *The Sopranos*. He's always coming home either way too late or way too early in the morning *not* to be cheating on Carmela. Check out *Brokeback Mountain* for indications your guy is leading a double life. *Sideways* isn't so much about wine as it is about the male psyche. Watch *Swingers* for clear insight into both the softer and the player side of guys. Likewise, check out *Gladiator* to see how an authentic man feels about the love of a woman. Look to *The Departed* to see both how a good yet complicated guy (Leonardo DiCaprio's character) views relationships with women and how a creep (Matt Damon's character) uses a woman as a front for his "good guy" image. Study male characters, ladies. You might find you know a lot about your guys.

Finally, if you figure out that he has nothing to offer you and that you're not learning anything (the entire premise of this book) or enjoying his company, he's probably using you emotionally. Get out. Get out if any of the items we've listed seem to proliferate in your relationship. Most important, don't feel used. Look at it both as an anthropological experiment—you now have your data to avoid this guy—and a learning experience that this guy mistook your kindness for weakness. To be kind and loving isn't a weakness, it's a strength. Be strong, walk away, and give your kindness and love to a man who reciprocates it in all ways.

How to End a Relationship

Lynne dated a guy named Justinian. He had a no-nonsense approach to all relationships. He told the women he dated exactly where he stood on male versus female communication styles, sex, love, and everything else that involves the differences between the sexes. One of the reasons Lynne loved hanging out with this guy (and still might) is because of his frank conversations with her about how he perceived women. He taught her about how most men perceived the differences between men and women and how they acted. He might not have been the first man who made Lynne realize she liked taking charge of her relationships much as men do, but he certainly brought her home on the issue. One cool February night they spent about an hour under the stars conversing about breakups and the fundamental difference between men and women on the topic.

"When you end the relationship, end it!" Justinian vehemently declared. "Don't call. Don't check in. Don't see how the other person is doing." That's it. Basically, it hurts too much on both sides to let it linger. For some reason, women try to remain "friends." It

When something reminds you of your ex-boyfriend, push it out of your mind. Otherwise, you might fall prey to this deadly trap of calling him and saying, "Remember when we used to watch *The Fresh Prince of Bel Air* together? I always think of you when I watch our show!" Then—too quickly—the guy with whom you broke up because he was a jerk and didn't treat you right invites you out. You go. You end up marrying him. You end up divorcing him, because he wasn't the right one. Call a friend instead of him and let the friend talk you out of calling the ex.

doesn't matter if you're separating after a twenty-year marriage or walking away from six weeks of fabulous fun that isn't going anywhere. It won't do either of you a bit of good to "check in." "What do you get to hear? That your ex is doing great without you?" asks Justinian. He makes the point that calling each other occasionally just prolongs the healing process. Too true. In fact, it isn't uncommon to find yourself in bed again with the person with whom you broke up.

Do you want to move on after the breakup? Good! Instead of spending relentless hours at the gym working on a body that'll bring him back or vomiting after crying for long hours, do what guys do. Go out. Pick up another guy. He's called the "transitional guy," and we highly recommend several transitional guys after the breakup. Nothing will take your mind off your ex sooner or better than the affection of someone delicious and new! This is the time, in fact, to date outside your regular "zone." Date older and younger men; guys who make less money and guys who make more than you; guys with and without facial hair; Socialists and Democrats; music lovers and bibliophiles; religious zealots and humanists. Date 'em all. Don't engage in relationships, just outings. (But if you sleep with any of them, we won't tell—wink-wink.)

What's the first thing a man's friends do after he breaks up? They take him clubbing or to a strip joint. *Break up and go out, girls.* That's our motto. Now is the perfect time to play the field.

How to Peacock: Displaying Your Assets

Trevor cycled 365 days a year. His chosen sport caused tremendous muscle development in his legs. Lynne hasn't dated anyone with calves as beautiful since her days cycling around Sacramento with this stud. Because he possessed such incredible lower limbs, Lynne loved the fact that he flaunted them, flagrantly wearing shorts year-round (not cycling shorts!). Soccer shorts, khakis, hiking shorts—it didn't matter. In the winter he wore shorts and long-sleeve shirts. Trevor claimed his legs were never cold, but really. The guy knew his best asset and he flaunted it. We all need to take a lesson from Trevor: show 'em what you got.

Ever look at the animal kingdom and notice that the male of the species always wears the more colorful outerwear? Look at the peacock. Males showcase beautiful hues of blue, black, and green, along with other shades in their feathers and literally parade in front of lady birds fully erect! Why do you think women wear makeup? It's our way of compensating for Mother Nature's lack of bright colors that entice the opposite sex.

As women, we're also nurtured to show modesty in all ways. We're initially taught to tone down our aggressiveness and cover up. We ask instead of tell. We're called sluts if we show a little skin. Certainly, you don't want your breasts hanging out at a business meeting, but what about a little cleavage when you're out shopping or running errands or meeting men? Show them what you got, sugar. At the same time, if your smile causes Jedi mind tricks, *smile*, for goodness' sake!

Fill in the blank: My best feature is _____.

Okay, now commit to making sure that at least one guy sees that asset each day—anyone from the letter carrier to the grocery clerk.

Why are we espousing flaunting your best features to the opposite sex? Because men do it all the time, with confidence. And ask anyone—confidence is the sexiest asset of them all!

How to Check Him Out Like He Checks You Out

Lynne loves checking out men from head to toe, especially without their noticing. And she's particularly proud of her ability to shamelessly leer at men. The first time she tried it was with a coworker. At a lunch meeting with about fifty colleagues, she became mesmerized as he sat next to her. She couldn't take her eyes off of his strong biceps, huge thigh muscles from years of playing professional sports, and huge, strong hands. She took him in like a tiger going after its prey. After the glance, she almost felt like she'd had sex. It was that good looking at him. Nothing came of it, though. It was just a beautiful moment and a feeling of power. A year later, Lynne caught a colleague looking at her and she called him on it. "Damn straight I was checking you out," he said. "I'll look if I want. You look hot in those boots." He didn't deny it, and this sent Lynne atwitter. From that day on, if she wanted to check out a man, she would. Here's how to do it without getting caught:

1. First, check out your surroundings. Can you get away with it? The only reason Lynne could check out the colleague at such a public affair was his proximity to her and the nature of the crowded room. Another meeting and no way! Are you in church? Probably shouldn't leer at anyone. Decide if you can properly and shamelessly take in your guy.

2. You can? Then begin. Start with his chest. Linger there a bit. Imagine your head resting there after sex!

3. Look back up to his face. Does he have a strong jaw? Great lips? Imagine his lips on yours for a second. If you must, bite your lip.

4. Let your gaze travel back down his arms and slowly linger on his hands. Imagine his hands around your bare waist.

5. Check out his goods. Quickly. If you're lucky, you might get an idea of his package. Do we really need to tell you why?

6. Go down his legs, lingering on your favorite areas. Imagine those legs on your legs.

7. Breathe in deeply and slowly exhale as you take in the whole picture.

8. Now go back to whatever you were doing.

How to Pick Up a Guy

Lynne used to sit passively by and wait for a guy to approach her—until recently after she studied males in public places and how they tried to pick her up. Jennifer prides herself on having the perfect pickup line, which she used before she was married. This lesson takes what we've both learned and gives you two easy lines to use to pick up a date. They worked for us both. Follow these steps to pick up any guy, any time:

1. Banish all fear. Guys learn early that they must push fear away in order to get the girl. In the hunt, one cannot move passively.

2. Make up your mind that you're going to talk first. Get ready to approach the guy.

3. Turn your head to him and smile. A smile actually disarms people, making them more accessible.

4. Jennifer's line: "Would you be shocked if I made a pass at you?" If he's at all interested, he'll make the pass. That's the beauty of Jennifer's line; she need not carry on from here. It's his job to continue the pickup. She's let him know she's interested.

5. Lynne's line: "You're not from around here, are you?" Invariably, the guy will quizzically answer her with a question, "Are you from around here?" They've launched into a conversation if he's at all interested.

6. Close the deal by asking, "Do you know of someplace quieter we can get a drink?" If he's interested, he'll suggest his place.

How to Move from Man to Man in the World of Hookup Dating without Bitterness

Lynne's friend Allison hasn't been divorced long. After a brief nuptial right out of high school and a child, she suddenly found herself out in the dating world with limited experience. She's young and didn't know how to navigate this new age of "hookups," as she'd only ever been with her high school sweetheart–turned-husband. Allison began going out with her girlfriends and couldn't get beyond the "hookup" mentality, the idea that people no longer dated and had relationships but instead hooked up for a night or two of physical encounters. Finally, she thought, "If I can't beat them, I'll join them." Allison decided to view each encounter as nothing more than sex with no expectations. She soon posted a profile on a dating Web site. She likes the anonymity of it all now and has "learned to use men the way they use women," a cavalier approach, indeed.

This book isn't about hookups, yet we need to address this phenomenon. The phrase "hooking up" connotes that the two parties involved engage in sexual activity for the pleasure of the moment and then move on to another sexual encounter. There is no permanency in the relationship and there are no expectations. If you expect a call from a guy after you've had sex, hookup sex probably isn't for you.

Truthfully, we don't like the idea of hooking up with one man after another. You don't learn anything from a guy if he's a one-night stand (well, perhaps some sexual moves but not the depth of knowledge relationships bring; even the sex gets better the more you're with someone).

We love men! We love nurturing relationships with them in which we both learn and teach. Truthfully, as much as you're learning from him, he's learning from you, too. All this learning and exchanging of fascinating experiences eludes you if you participate in the hookup world. We love spending time with men over and over until we decide to move on. Look at *Sex and the City*. Carrie and the girls might have hooked up quite a few times, but they only really learned from the consistent relationships and were looking for a strong bond with a man, not a few minutes of meaningless, unsatisfying physical connections.

So the question remains, how do you hook up with man after man without any bitterness? We address this pretty succinctly in the section When to Sleep with a Guy (page 156). It comes down to this:

- If you want to avoid bitterness, do only what makes you comfortable. Think critically about what you can live with. Will you be okay bumping into a guy you hooked up with the previous Friday if you are now out with his friend? Or conversely, if he's out with one of your girlfriends?

- Truth is, we still live in a patriarchal society that approves of men having numerous sexual partners. But women are still called "pass around" or "sluts" if they choose this lifestyle. So if you choose it, make sure you don't care about what people say. Look at each hookup as pleasure you received—nothing more, nothing less.

- Lynne's friend Allison made a conscious decision not to become attached to any man with whom she slept, going so far as to only hook up through Internet sites based entirely on this premise. She doesn't want the complications that exist with an emotional connection. We love the emotional and mental idea of a relationship, whether it lasts a few weeks or a few years. You need to decide what's right for you.

- Decide if this is going to be a lifestyle or just a "sample" phase. Maybe you're curious about the concept of sexual free- dom. You might not see yourself as a serial hookup propo- nent, but as someone who'd like to experience a more sexually adventurous side. Maybe you're coming out of a long-term relationship and the idea of no-commitment sex sounds great. We can't stress, enough, however, that *you need to know what you can live with.* If you decide to live the hookup lifestyle, don't expect a call. In fact, don't give out your phone number and don't ask for his, because that's the whole idea—no commitment past each encounter. You must have a cavalier attitude about sex to make this work.

If you follow these steps and expect nothing more than one hookup after another, you won't find yourself bitter. But again, we must end by saying, *Boyfriend University* isn't about hookups; it's about relationships. What you can learn and take on to build a successful career and love life. Hookups aren't about building relationships, so what's the fun beyond a few primal minutes? It might have its place, but it's not a good way to empower oneself with much knowledge—even sexual knowledge comes with building a relationship. Finally, if you engage in this aspect of the new millennium's sexual revolution, make sure to use a condom.

Cheat Sheet: Sex Rules and Information— from Kissing to Foreplay to Fantasies

Just as a teacher doesn't necessarily pull all the test questions from one chapter, not all the relationship tips we've learned at Boyfriend University fit into one specific section. This is sort of a catchall section, offering concise tips on a variety of subjects we've picked up along the dating road that have served us well over the years. Have fun with these factoids both in the bedroom and out of it. Just don't get caught and earn yourself an indecent exposure rap!

KISSING

Everyone we talked to—male and female—has tales of kissing woe and wonder. Jennifer likens kissing one younger man to "being blanketed in clouds." Liz, Lynne's friend, tells the horror story of the "pointy-tongued, condorlike kisser." Ick! Nevertheless, here are the best tips we found for kissing:

- If you don't like the way he kisses you, gently tell him what you like. School him in your kissing ideals—he won't mind at all. If you like a more gentle approach than his shoving his tongue violently down your throat, let him know. If you prefer a rougher edge, let him know that, too. If that doesn't

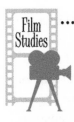

Film Studies

Get yourself in the kissing mood. Navigate to YouTube and search for the last scene of *Cinema Paradiso* or type in this link: www .youtube.com/watch?v=wEFugVbzsSo. What follows is film history and the sexiest few minutes of screen kisses ever cut together.

work, you'll have to actually show him what you like. It's a good bet he'll follow your lead and move like you do. If he doesn't follow your lead, tell him to sit back and enjoy the kisses. Kiss him everywhere and in all ways that you want to be kissed, then tell him to duplicate it on you!

- We mentioned it in the section How to Hide Bad Behavior (page 150), but it bears repeating: if you're the other woman, don't teach him new kissing tricks. Don't be naive. The way he kisses you is the way he kisses his wife (and he does kiss his wife). If you teach him a new way to kiss, she'll clue in to the extramarital activities, squelching your fun.

- Always keep a toothbrush and toothpaste in your purse. Kissing a sour mouth is the worst! Ever kiss a guy whose mouth is sour from too much booze and you'll know what we mean. You want to make sure your breath is kissing fresh!

- Spend a day kissing every inch of his body. You'd be surprised where he discovers he likes the kisses.

- Lots of lipstick is usually a turnoff, ladies. Tone it down and go for the clearer glosses when you'll spend the night smacking lips. One exception: put on red lipstick and turn him on by leaving lip prints down his belly and lower. Hot!

- A hard, forceful tongue never works. The more relaxed your tongue in the French-kissing process, the more pleasure. Ease up.

- Give the guy two kissing chances. If he isn't a good kisser the first go-round, try again. Lynne dated a guy who gave her the most forceful, aggressive good-night kisses on their first date. They were okay, but not great. She didn't go out with him for four more months, finally letting his lips touch hers again. Guess what? *Voilà, mon amie!* He kissed her with amazing ease, strength, and sex appeal. Wow! What if she didn't give him the second chance? A guy might be nervous his first time kissing you. Give him a chance to redeem himself. If he doesn't improve, move on. Don't let a bird of prey continue to peck at you!

- Smooching is personalized. You feel your way into it during this gig. Relax and enjoy. If you give robotic kisses, he'll head for a less mechanical kissing adventure.

- Public kissing isn't taboo. Public mauling is. When you kiss in public, don't necessarily open wide. Slightly parted lips and a little tongue works best. See the Film Studies sidebar on page 171 for more info.

PUT YOUR KNOWLEDGE TO WORK

Ever wanted to kiss a guy who seems too shy to make the first move? Jennifer and Lynne have. Lynne's ex-husband sat next to her on their first date, and it seemed obvious he was into her, but he wasn't making any moves—beyond a cursory hand on the leg occasionally as he leaned in to talk. Well, guess what, girls? If a guy touches you anywhere on your body—arm, leg, shoulder—even if momentarily, that's your big sign that he's open to a kiss. He wouldn't touch you if he didn't want to kiss you. Lynne took the sign and leaned over delicately, kissing him on the cheek. She pulled away slowly, slowly enough for him to plant a kiss on her lips. They spent the next hour in the car making out!

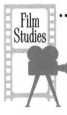

Film Studies

In *The Wedding Singer*, with Adam Sandler and Drew Barrymore, Barrymore's character tries to explain to her cousin how she will kiss her husband at the altar. In one of the more hilarious descriptions of French kissing on camera, she says, "Not porno tongue, church tongue." Her cousin insists on seeing what church tongue is. "It's mouth slightly opened, some tongue," Barrymore replies.

TRICKS

Believe it or not, men's egos are fragile yet *big*. They like to believe that no one has ever been in bed with you before them. Jennifer tells a great story about hooking up with a guy she dated for one last liaison in the bedroom. She pulled her signature sex move, a little hot trick she regularly used, and the former boyfriend said after his ecstasy, "I can't believe you remembered how to do that for me." Funny. He thought she'd done it for him and only for him. She could have told him the truth, but why? If you have a trick, let him think it's only for him.

Try to remember your signature moves that you've used and haven't used on guys. Lynne had an uncomfortable moment with a lover whom she reacquainted herself with one evening. She kissed him someplace she could have sworn he loved. Not so much! "I thought you loved that!" she exclaimed. "Uh, no, must not have been me," he said. Awkward. Lesson: shut up if he's not that enthused about the move. It might not have been *his* favorite in your arsenal of sex tricks.

MUSIC TO MOVE YOU

Music moves the soul and the body. Who can deny the power music holds over us? Here's a list of ten pieces from ten very different artists that are certain to set your bodies in sweet motion.

These are sexy tunes, not romantic ones, and it certainly isn't a complete list, but it will get you started:

1. Maurice Ravel, "Bolero"
2. AC/DC, "You Shook Me All Night Long"
3. Tricky, "Suffocated Love"
4. Prince, "I Wanna Be Your Lover"
5. Marvin Gaye, "Sexual Healing"
6. Godsmack, "Voodoo"
7. Bryan Ferry, "Slave to Love"
8. Dave Matthews Band, "Crash"
9. Divinyls, "I Touch Myself"
10. Fiona Apple, "Shadowboxer"

TEN SEX RULES AND CLUES

These ten items detail a few things to consider regarding sex in our world. Some deal with the age-old question of fidelity, others look at more modern viewpoints. They're just a few of the things we learned that have made us wiser and better in relationships.

1. If he never lets you sleep at his place, he's probably a cheater. If your guy always has sex at your place, dump him.
2. Don't let anyone do anything to you that makes you uncomfortable. Any man who forces you to have sex is a rapist, not a boyfriend. All good guys swear this to be true!
3. If he never calls you, he's not interested.
4. Not all men necessarily like the new rage of the Brazilian wax. Some men prefer a few more leaves on their bush. You'll need to investigate.

5. Part of empowering yourself in relationships means not settling for just anyone. Only date men who make you feel good about yourself and whom you'd proudly introduce to anyone. If you're ashamed of him, he's not the right one. Even if the sex is great—for now—you'll begin to resent him even in bed the more you see the loser. Don't let yourself get to the stage of having to toss back a stiff drink before bed. Dump him.

6. Use protection, no matter how old you are. First, safe sex remains a must in this day and age. Next, getting pregnant isn't fair to anyone if one party isn't ready or doesn't want to be a parent. If the man refuses protection, be wary, very wary. In fact, don't sleep with him.

7. Animals have no rules regarding sex. If you decide to go animal, don't follow rules. Let the wild kingdom rule you.

8. Role playing, sex toys, and adventurous positions can all prove exciting in the bedroom, but only within your and his comfort zones. The *Kama Sutra*, for example, might find you in bedded bliss, while fuzzy, pink handcuffs might find you running from the bedroom!

9. Never settle for a sexless relationship unless it's for spiritual reasons. If a man insists you're his girlfriend or wife but doesn't want to make love to you, he's playing around or just plain strange. Remember, Maslow's Hierarchy of Needs lists sex as a must for survival. You deserve the pleasure of sex.

10. If he pleasures you, pleasure him in return. This is a team sport, ladies, not an individual race.

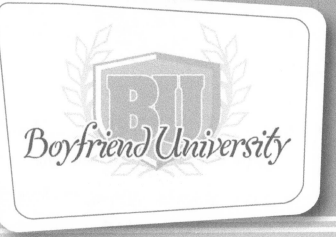

Extracurriculars

There are those men who are less concerned with academics than with the partying associated with university life. This part covers the information gleaned from men who look upon life as a big playground.

9

Studying Abroad

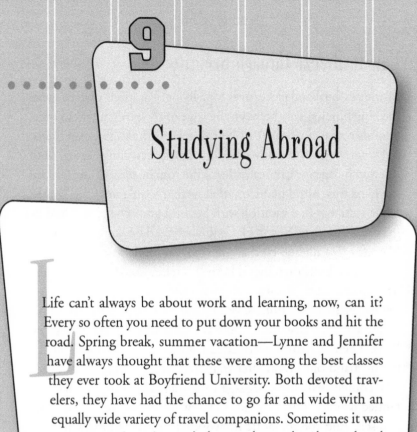

Life can't always be about work and learning, now, can it? Every so often you need to put down your books and hit the road. Spring break, summer vacation—Lynne and Jennifer have always thought that these were among the best classes they ever took at Boyfriend University. Both devoted travelers, they have had the chance to go far and wide with an equally wide variety of travel companions. Sometimes it was great, sometimes it wasn't, but as always they learned and are now ready to share that knowledge with you. From learning to navigate city streets or assess the changing weather conditions, they picked up skills that will help you in all of your journeys.

Traveling can be a wonderful way to get to know someone. Traveling on your own can be a wonderful way to meet someone. Taking a trip can also be the death knell for a relationship that was never going to go anywhere anyway, so you might as well heed the signs and get it over with. We'll even help you decide if your travel companion needs to be tossed overboard.

How to Breeze through Security

Lynne's ex-husband globe-trots for a living. Vacations used to mean meeting him halfway between the edge of the earth and her home. Sounds romantic, doesn't it? Nothing beats the sunset over Siena, Italy, with a man you love. Unfortunately, traveling abroad with too much baggage can really derail the romance, as Lynne learned the hard way. She'd never traveled farther than across the United States until her first vacation with her husband. The plan? She'd fly from California to New York City, where he'd booked a suite at the Plaza for two nights. He'd arrive from an undisclosed location in the Middle East, then they'd both fly to Europe for fourteen days of touring. Ludicrously, Lynne packed for fourteen days and nights. First, items from sexy lingerie to stiletto heels to crystal wineglasses got lost somewhere between the United States and Paris. Then, her three overloaded bags were lugged unhappily by her husband onto train after train and along cobblestone streets. The couple's expensive luggage took such a beating that its warrantied handles actually broke. Oh how her guy cursed! He was not amused. And the romantic fireworks? Defused. To make matters worse, while her husband breezed through security, Lynne seemed to get frisked at every border crossing.

Men know how to swiftly pass through security, laptop ready for scanning, tickets and passport snugly in suit pocket. What can you learn from them about how to get through security easily, catch your plane calmly, and leave unnecessary luggage behind? A lot! Lynne no longer carries crystal on trips abroad (when you're in love, who cares whether the champagne flutes are Waterford or glass?) and can get all her belongings into one backpack or bag. Now's your turn to see how it's done.

CHECK YOUR EGO WITH THE LUGGAGE

As much as we and most other women would love to share real estate with David Beckham, we don't live the "Posh" lifestyle when traveling. We have no makeup artist sitting next to us in first class; no beds on transcontinental flights; no bodyguards carrying twenty bags of shoes, clothes, and accessories from England to Spain to the United States and then back.

What's this mean? Check your ego with the luggage, honey. Most men on vacation don't worry about paparazzi and therefore don't worry about how they look on the plane. Forget about makeup and high heels, tight skirts and fishnet hose. Think clean and comfortable. Get rid of, or at the very least limit, all accessories.

One former boyfriend of Lynne's actually wore soccer shorts, a T-shirt, and flip-flops on all flights. He doesn't look like the cover of *GQ*, but Jeremy sails through security. Nothing blips, beeps, or yelps when he passes under the security monitors.

A good guy pal of Lynne's does the same thing but for a different reason. Stan has a metal rod in his leg. He knows security will go off when he walks through the metal detectors. Without any watch, belt, or shoes to mess with, he might get stopped but won't juggle the junk and waste even more time getting through security.

So, ladies, follow their lead. Banish the dangling earrings, the Brighton bracelets, the sexy stilettos with the steel, dominatrix toe, and the jeweled belt. Throw on a pair of cute Juicy sweats and flip-flops.

NEVER TAKE YOUR LAPTOP ON VACATION

Come on, it's break time. We certainly hope you're doing something better than checking your MySpace account while new sights, cities, and men await you. Only when he's on a business trip does a man lug a laptop.

You're a girl, so you'll probably carry a purse unless you've purchased a handy laptop/tote bag. Why carry essentially two purses, one of which is extra heavy with hardware? If you really must check e-mail, any self-respecting man-about-many-towns will tell you Internet cafés exist everywhere. Most hotels also provide a computer or two that travelers may log onto for a small fee.

CARRY AS LITTLE AS POSSIBLE ONTO THE AIRCRAFT

Yes, we women love our purses because they hold things. But what things do you really need to have in those purses on a plane? Especially now with security so tight, who doesn't have a friend whose favorite lip gloss or hand cream got confiscated? Lynne remembers when she'd carry her purse full of toiletries and a makeup box on the

Do you know the rules regarding liquids on aircraft? Do you realize what security screeners might take from you if you don't follow the rules? To find out exactly how many ounces of what you're allowed to carry on your flight, navigate to www.tsa.gov. You'll find everything from lists of prohibited items to tips for traveling with kids. As of this writing, liquids, gels, and aerosols must be three ounces or less. And no sharp objects, either. Yep, no tweezers!

plane, so she could literally clean up in the plane bathroom and completely redo her makeup and even, yes, hair before landing. Not today. All of her jars and tubes would end up in a Department of Transportation or Homeland Security bin before she could pass her E-ticket to the attendant at boarding.

POSSESS A DESIGNATED POUCH OR POCKET

When it comes to your tickets, passport, other identification, visas, and money, have one pocket or pouch in a purse (or, as ugly as this sounds, a fanny pack) that is purposely dedicated to these items.

You'll need to pull them out and keep them out in long security lines. Just as guys line up all their tools, on trips they tend to line up all their important documentation and money. Whereas we gals might carry a cute tote with crevices and nooks and crannies, it screws us up in security. Do yourself a favor and dump most everything out of your purse (including all those old receipts, the electric bill, and the extra twenty lip balms). Then assign one pocket to your important travel documentation and identification.

Finally, have fun. Look at the airport as an adventure. Lynne's former flame Stev says he looks forward to the endless possibilities of a new relationship at an airport. "Who knows who is leaving whom and might be on your plane? You might meet the person of your dreams on a Boeing 747 heading to Boulder, Colorado." You never know, but if you're too busy digging for your identification and trying to throw all your jewelry through the scanner, you won't be looking up to see your soul mate!

How to Explore a Foreign City and Find Your Way Back to the Hotel

Erik Devonic jumped from airplanes, scuba dived, scaled walls, and hit the beach in faraway lands. Adventure was his modus operandi—in both his work and his play. Travel, therefore, played an integral part when Lynne dated "Dev."

Dev knew how to get around and find his way back. From him, Lynne learned how to leave the hotel, explore a foreign city by foot, and not worry at all about finding her way back—sans compass and map—to a hot bubble bath and a rich Chianti. She has confidently canvassed local streets and foreign cities with equal success, never fearing she wouldn't find her way home. Here's what you need to know about land navigation.

START BY PLANNING NOT TO GET LOST

The most important part of land navigation and exploring a foreign place is planning. You don't just begin walking without thinking. Follow these tips and you'll always know where you are, or at least where you should be:

- If you have a compass, carry it. Compasses are small and come in handy if you really don't know what direction you're traveling. Let's say you leave the hotel and begin walking southbound according to the compass. By heading north when you're ready to return, you'll be moving in the right direction.

- If you have a map, use it. Begin by finding your location on the map. Take note of the streets surrounding your location and the directions they traverse—north, south, east, west. Here's where your orientation will especially work in conjunction with a compass.

PUT YOUR KNOWLEDGE TO WORK

You're attending a business seminar in a large city. All of your colleagues and your boss will be there. No one knows the town at all. Between breakout sessions, get to know the town and the surrounding area. Using your land-navigation skills, you may stumble upon a quaint bistro or a cool pub. Day two of the conference, wow your coworkers by suggesting everyone take a jaunt to the hip and delicious restaurant you found or the fabulous antiques market. Your boss will most likely find your initiative commendable and your fellow office mates may just end up with a fantastic feast. (Doesn't most conference food lack taste? Who wants another course of rubbery chicken Cordon Bleu?) For weeks everyone will talk about how the great adventure they took with you at the helm helped alleviate the boredom of the conference!

- If you don't have a compass or a map, ask the concierge for landmarks in the general vicinity. What's out there? Take Rome, for example, a city Lynne has explored on her own. She knew that surrounding her hotel within a five-mile radius were the Coliseum, Piazza Navona, the Roman Forum, Castel St. Angelo, and more. She had an idea of the area before she trotted off. Granted, she didn't know exactly where everything was—but she knew that if she was at the Coliseum, she was just a few miles from the hotel.

- Know what your home base looks like both coming and going. It's a concept every member of the military knows. Look at your surroundings as you are leaving, making a mental note of the landmarks, street names, and buildings. But also look at those surroundings from the perspective of returning. What does the place look like walking to it from the street? Things look different depending on whether you're coming or going. If you know what your environment looks like coming, you'll recognize it more easily upon your return.

Extra Credit

Sometimes no matter how well you navigate, you get lost. It happens to the best of us. But instead of taking a cue from your dad on that family car trip and *not* asking directions, go ahead and ask for help. Typically, you'll find you're not as lost as you may have thought. Hide your pride and find some help. It may save you hours of frustration.

- Take a mental note of interesting markers—a quaint restaurant, a cutting-edge clothing store, an attention-grabbing monument—along your march. On her tour of Rome, for example, Lynne noted the Egyptian obelisk near the hotel. Even a strange-looking tree can act as a marker. Hansel and Gretel had bread crumbs; you have landmarks.

- Know what time it is. If you've been meandering east for an hour, meandering west for another hour should find you close to your starting point.

- Know your abilities. If you aren't used to walking miles upon miles, don't explore for two hours and then expect to have an easy walk back for another two hours. You'll be exhausted and blistered.

Dev left Lynne with one more great piece of advice: always take two days to really explore. Use the first day to just walk around practicing your land navigation. On the second day, you'll have a better feel for the environment and can go back and investigate areas that piqued your interest.

> **Extra Credit**
> We highly recommend fearlessly exploring foreign lands, but only when you're in a reasonably safe town. Don't go promenading, for example, in Bogotá, Colombia. Before you plan an excursion, check with the State Department. Although most places are safe to walk around, there are certain areas that really shouldn't be explored, depending upon the country. One wrong turn and you could find yourself in a deadly situation. Use your gut, your brain, and your prudence when deciding whether to trek out of bounds.

How to Fathom a Street Grid

In college Jennifer got a job as a pizza delivery person in Berkeley, California. So naturally she began dating the manager. After a few nights of Jennifer's wandering aimlessly around the streets in her little car, trying hard to find various addresses and buildings, he taught her how to understand a numbering grid and a few lessons in basic city design. All became clear, and she not only delivered pizzas while they were still hot, but she is also completely at ease in almost any big city. Once you understand what all those street numbers mean, the world is your oyster.

Most cities and towns didn't spring up out of nowhere. First someone decided, "Great place to build a town. It is right next to a river [big rock, shady tree, railroad track, whatever]." The town then developed slowly over time and a few streets were built. Sometimes the townspeople named the streets after the alphabet—A Street, B Street, and so on. Sometimes they called them by numbers—First Street, Second Street, and so on. How did they decide which would be A Street, or First Street? Probably by starting next to the very thing that drew them to the area (river, big rock, shady tree, railroad track). So in almost every town, if there is a First Street or an A Street, you can bet it sits next to a river and that the streets flow from there. In Berkeley, where Jennifer delivered her pizzas, First Street is at the edge of town right next to the San Francisco Bay. In Sacramento, where she grew up, First Street runs north and south and is next to the Sacramento River, and A Street runs east and west and is next to the American River. See how that works? So if you are ever looking for a small numbered street, or a street toward the beginning of the alphabet, it is a good guess to head toward a river.

Another important thing to know when wandering around a neighborhood trying to find a particular address is that even-numbered houses are on one side of the street, and odd-numbered houses are on the other. They are never, ever mixed. Sure, you probably already knew this, but Jennifer did not until she started driving around at night with pizza in the car, peering in the dark at strange houses.

In any town laid out on a grid system, you need to familiarize yourself with the addresses as they intersect with a few major streets, and that will help you navigate. Every New Yorker knows

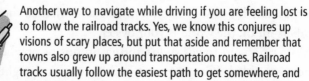

Another way to navigate while driving if you are feeling lost is to follow the railroad tracks. Yes, we know this conjures up visions of scary places, but put that aside and remember that towns also grew up around transportation routes. Railroad tracks usually follow the easiest path to get somewhere, and most main roads more or less follow them. If you find a railroad track and follow it, you are likely to get somewhere important pretty soon. Just don't ever walk on railroad tracks. Too many tragic deaths occur each year as the result of people walking on tracks.

that Fifth Avenue divides the addresses in New York from east to west, so an address that is, say, 15 West Fifty-seventh Street is literally just steps away from the intersection of Fifth Avenue and West Fifty-seventh. Most other towns have a quirk like that that will help you learn your way around. In Berkeley, where she hasn't lived in years, Jennifer remembers that the 2500 block of any north-to-south street crosses the east-west street at Dwight Avenue, so she can still look at an address and know pretty much where the building is. Take the time to memorize the address at the major intersection of your town (or the places you visit often) and you, too, can demystify a street grid system.

How to Find the North Star

Why would you want to find the North Star, anyway? What good will that info do you? If you can find the North Star, then should you ever find yourself lost in the woods you will be able to know which way is south, west, and east. Then you can decide to walk whichever way strikes your fancy. Hopefully you will head toward where you think civilization will be found.

To find the North Star, first look up. Okay, that does sound silly, but it is a first step. And don't look too far up, not to the top of the sky, but just about a quarter of the way up from the horizon. Now, can you find the Big Dipper? Remember where that is? The North Star, also called Polaris, actually stays stable, while the Big Dipper rotates around it throughout the year. That is why sailors used it as, well, the North Star.

So the North Star must really be north, right, hanging there in the sky directly over the North Pole? No. A cool factoid to use someday to impress someone is that the North Star is actually one degree off north.

Find the Big Dipper and draw an imaginary line straight out from the two stars that are at the end of the bowl, the actual dipper part. That imaginary line will lead you to the Little Dipper, and there it is—the North Star. The North Star itself is actually part of the Little Dipper; it is the very last star on the handle.

10

Spring Break and Summer Vacation

Life cannot be all work. Why do you think spring break remains a hallowed week in our world? When we play, we rejuvenate ourselves to get back into the real world. This section offers lessons that'll not only teach you fun activities but also show you how to get out of a bind.

How to Plan the Perfect Weekend

Sometimes the trips that you anticipate the longest can be the biggest letdowns. They have existed in your mind for so long as perfect, that once you are actually at the hotel you longed to visit you notice how shabby the carpet is and that the beach isn't quite as fab as you expected and the whole place makes you sad. On the other hand, sometimes the trips you didn't anticipate at all—the last-minute dash out of town or the extra ticket to Paris a friend offers— leave the greatest impression. Jennifer once turned to her boyfriend Cub and said, "Let's take Sherry with us the next time we go to Mexico. She's never been." He nodded solemnly and said, "Tell her we'll pick her up tonight at ten." And off they went to Baja California for the weekend on the spur of the moment. Jennifer can still recall everything they did on that wild road trip.

Yes, sometimes the perfect weekend involves no planning. Whether you are traveling on your own on some grand adventure, or with a lover, or a friend, the best trips can be those that unfold on their own. But how do you plan a weekend trip without planning? Like this:

Choose a weekend. We don't want you to plan, but you need to at least determine a few days where you won't be missed at work, or needed around the house. And if this is a trip with a lover, you need to make sure he can get away then, too. So go ahead and choose a date.

PUT YOUR KNOWLEDGE TO **WORK**

If you do have a travel destination in mind, we recommend that you don't spend a whole lot of time reading travel magazines. Why not? Because they might set you up for disappointment when you actually arrive at the real place. Nothing is ever as perfect as it is in a magazine photo. Instead, read books that are set in the place you want to visit. Novels, history books, biographies, travel accounts, anything that will help you know the place when you get there and give you an additional way to look at what is around you. *Hey! Isn't that where the last battle took place? Over there, isn't that where Marlena met her Italian count? And I think this little forest is where the children hid out during the storm.* Wouldn't that kind of knowledge be so much more interesting than, *Hey! There's that Starbuck's I read about.*

Choose a direction. North? South? East? West? Why not write them down on four small scraps of paper and draw one out of a hat.

Choose a travel method. Train? Car? Plane? Bike? Bus? Pick one that appeals, or use the small scraps of paper in a hat method for this part, too.

Choose a theme. A search for fresh seafood? The hunt for an antique desk? Immersing yourselves in nature? Choose a big theme that will help you shape your weekend once you arrive at wherever you are going.

Ready, set, go! Once you've chosen those four things, you are good to go. Don't spend time obsessing over the perfect destination hotels and room availability; it will all work out. Really, it will. The best weekend trips are spontaneous and free-form, and taking off without much of a plan will really let you get to know someone else. You might learn that you'd like to spend a lot more time with him, or you might learn that you never, ever, ever want to see him again.

The perfect weekend getaway should always involve food, don't you think? We do. But we would again caution against traveling with a long list of places you read about in the food section that you just have to go to. Imagine the heartache and frustration when the fantastic burger joint you had your heart set on turns out to be closed for the winter, or the chef who opened a tiny soup place couldn't pay his bills and skipped out in the middle of the night. Jennifer once traveled to the groovy town of Booneville, California, to eat in a place where the chef had done exactly that! So she is just trying to protect you from feeling the same disappointment. The better food approach is to follow your nose. Stand on the sidewalk and let yourself be seduced by the smell of cinnamon rolls; you'll find where it's coming from easily enough.

Always ask a local where you should eat. Locals will know exactly where to find the best burger, the biggest draft beer selection, the crispiest fries, and the driest martinis. And you will make a friend. Talking to people about food is always an easy way to break the ice; try it the next time you are on your own out of town and there is a handsome man nearby. "I was wondering, could you recommend a good place to find homemade apple pie?" Perhaps he will go out for pie with you.

How to Pack a Car for a Long Trip

While Jennifer was camping through Mexico's Baja peninsula some years ago, the back of her red Chevy Blazer was a wonder to behold, breathtakingly beautiful in its organization. Of course she didn't pack it herself. A very organized boyfriend did.

Knowing how to pack can make the difference between getting off to a good start to your road trip and standing screaming in frustration in the driveway of your house hours after you meant to leave. Which do you want to do? Right, you want to leave on time. Lucky for you, Jennifer was closely watching her boyfriend pack the Blazer and taking mental notes and can now tell you just how to do it. So here is how to pack a car for a long trip.

First, bring out everything that you plan to bring on the trip. Everything. Big stuff, small stuff—bring it all out and put it in the driveway or next to the street. If you have to pack your car out in public, you might want to have a minder who does nothing but watch to make sure that passersby don't pretend to think that you are giving away your possessions and help themselves to your stuff. If it is up to you to pack and keep an eye on your things at the same time, you won't do a good job at either.

If you skip this basic bring-it-all-out-first step and just haul out your things one at a time and put them into the back of the car in no particular order, the chances are big that you won't be able to fit everything. It's also likely that you might forget something important and it won't occur to you until you are miles away in another state.

Once you have everything that you plan to pack (remember, everything) out and near the car, give yourself a few minutes to just stand and look at it all. See if you can see anything you don't really need. See if you forgot something you really do need. See if there are any big things that can be condensed in any way, large, hard-sided objects that fit together like puzzle pieces in order to take up less room. Can you fit your suitcase inside the legs of the coffee table you are delivering to a friend? Give it a try.

Begin to pack the larger, stiffer things like hard-sided suitcases and boxes. Not only do these big things need to fit in first, but they are also the things you won't need until you arrive and won't have to have accessible during the drive. Put in your tent, your metal trunk, that coffee table, and whatever else is huge. Once you have the large pieces situated, start to fill up space with soft-sided things like sleeping bags, canvas suitcases, sports bags, sweaters and coats, and extra shoes.

PUT YOUR KNOWLEDGE TO WORK

Once you know how to pack a car, what else can you do with this skill? Hmm . . . reorganize your closets, perhaps? Fit more in your rented storage unit than you ever thought possible? You'll certainly know how to quickly fill up a moving van should you ever decide to leave town.

Always make sure that the things you might need during the day on your road trip are easy to get to—snow chains, maps, towels, or your lunch.

Packing for a big road trip is no time to get nervous. Chances are you will forget something, but so what? Don't panic; that's part of the adventure. If it's really important, you can typically pick it up at your destination—unless, of course, you're driving someplace like Kathmandu!

How to Get Along on the Open Road

Jennifer has logged many thousands of miles on the open road, first with her parents and siblings as they cruised the country from end to end, then with boyfriends as they raced up and down the length of the West Coast, headed sometimes for Canada, sometimes for Mexico. She loves to drive—the longer the distance, the better.

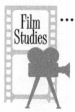

Film Studies

Want to check out a beautiful, mystical, and romantic road trip from the big screen? Rent *Elizabethtown*, starring Kirsten Dunst and Orlando Bloom. Curl up and enjoy it on your small screen.

There are rules for road trips. Jennifer didn't know that until one man firmly laid his road trip rule out for her: "I'm the driver. So I get to choose the music. When it's your turn to drive, it's your turn to choose the music." Seemed fair enough. Over the years she has learned the other rules that apply when you and a man hit the road together:

- **Music.** Yes, it is true that the driver gets to choose the music. Come prepared with a selection of your own tunes; don't rely on his bringing along what you like to hear in the middle of the night on a desert road when you are at the wheel.

- **Food.** Make sure you both agree on whether snacking in the car is allowed. Some men freak if you eat in their cars; others treat their own cars like large trash cans and you might be the one who freaks.

- **Climate control.** Unless the car has dual heating and cooling systems, you will need to work with each other to strike a happy medium between who is too cold and who is too hot. Avoid one of those silly scenes where you are each reaching over to turn it on, then off, then on again. Speak up and work it out. If you need to bring along a lap blanket in order to stay warm, do it.

- **Bathroom stops.** In fact, there are no rules about bathroom stops. If you need to go, he stops, and vice versa. If you're ever with a man who tells you there are rules about how often he will stop for the bathroom, drop him.

- **Conversation.** Sure, it is nice to talk as the miles roll by, but sitting together in silence is a big part of a road trip. Look out the window, read a book, knit a sweater, study the map. No one likes to be stuck in a car with a motormouth, and if he is the one who is chatting endlessly away, suggest kindly that it is time for quiet meditation on the scenery around you.

- **Money.** Decide in advance how you are going to deal with money for gas and food. Splitting it is always a fair deal, unless you are accompanying him on a trip he needed to make anyway. And if he has "forgotten" to bring his wallet along (it has happened to us, and we bet it has happened to you!), then this is probably the last time you are getting in a car with the man.

- **Conflict.** The car is not a good place to fight, so try to stay away from any subjects that you know will start you both up. Think about it: you can't walk off in a huff if you are stuck in the car next to him, and you also don't want to get into one of those scary situations where some angry person is behind the wheel of thousands of pounds of steel.

● **Cars.** Whose do you take? Whichever one will get the best gas mileage, has up-to-date insurance and registration, and has two working seat belts.

Having spent so much time on the road, there are four kinds of places we highly recommend you stop at whenever you get the chance:

1. **Oddball museums.** We mean places like the Barbed Wire Museum in LaCrosse, Kansas, or Leila's Hair Museum in Independence, Missouri. You can find weird museums in every state by checking out the listings at www.thetwinetour.com.

2. **Specialty factories offering tours.** Yes, you know you want to take the Jelly Belly factory tour, don't you? It'll give you a chance to fill your pockets with chewy jelly beans of all colors. How can you resist? Jennifer showed up late on the first day of graduate school because her boyfriend Cub wanted to tour a Wonder Bread factory. Find a tour near you at www.factorytoursusa.com.

3. **Used bookstores.** You just never know what you might stumble across in a used bookstore, and it isn't always a book. Art, music, collectibles—all manner of things are there to be found. And the coolest people work at used bookstores, so be sure and ask them about their town. You may quickly hear about a CD-release party, an all-night rave, or a beach bonfire that is taking place nearby.

4. **Outdoor markets.** Open-air farmers' markets are everywhere now, and if you stumble across one on your road trips you should always pull over and check it out. Homemade tamales, fresh strawberries, and locally grown, vine-ripened tomatoes are just some of the treasures you'll find. Beats stopping for a fast-food burger anytime. Markets are also a great source of info on what is happening in an area, so let people know you are from out of town and open to their suggestions.

- **Packing.** Make sure to read the lesson we included on the best way to pack a car; it will help you keep things nice and neat on the road. You don't want to have to haul your stuff out in a parking lot every time you need something from your suitcase. And you don't need to bring along every little thing; neither does he. Pack light, keep the car tidy, and you will both be happier.

- **Extra stops.** Other than bathroom stops (for which there are no rules), is there something that you always, always stop for? Jennifer always stops for signs that say "Homemade Pie," and Lynne keeps an eye out for community rummage sales. And maybe he always stops at motorcycle shops. Whatever your pleasure, let your travel companion know about it in advance so that no one gripes when you suddenly pull over.

- **Phone calls and texting.** You are in the car together, so don't spend your whole trip texting friends and chatting on your phone. Practice the Zen-like philosophy of being in the now.

Keep these rules in mind and your road trip will go smoothly. It's best to discuss all of the above before you even back the car out of the driveway.

How to Be Brave When Necessary

When spelunking (exploring underground caves) with her friend Sherry, Jennifer turned to her and said, "What we are about to do will probably be really scary and dangerous, but let's just not talk about that until it is over." And it worked. By focusing their energy on having fun instead of being scared, Jennifer and Sherry climbed without safety harnesses and shimmied through dark and narrow holes as if they'd been doing it for years. Sometimes life puts us in pretty scary and dangerous situations. Sometimes men put themselves in pretty scary and dangerous situations on purpose. What are they thinking?

It is important to know that your body will be there when you need it to be. That is what adrenaline is for. Nature has designed it so that when you are under attack, or in need of extra strength, it comes through in astonishing ways. You've heard those stories of mothers who lift cars off their children, or women who fight their way to freedom in dire circumstances. It happens because of adrenaline.

Here's a bravery trick: check your reactions with someone who has been through this before. If the pros aren't nervous about what is happening, then you shouldn't be, either. Some years back Jennifer was on a boat going from Sweden to England. Although she has logged a fair amount of time sailing around on small boats, she hasn't been on ocean crossings that often and, well, it seemed a bit rough to her. Like, really, really rough. A big storm was tossing the ship back and forth in a way that was pretty dang scary. She was terrified, not feeling brave at all, until she thought of a way to reassure herself. Getting up out of her narrow little bunk, she dressed and went to the bar. Her theory was that if it was business as usual in the bar that night, if the people who actually worked on the boat and made this crossing all the time seemed pretty calm, then it must be okay. Sure enough, the bartenders and waitresses didn't look at all nervous about what was happening, so she decided the storm wasn't that bad and the boat was not in fact

> **Extra Credit**
> Know when to be brave, but also know when to say no. Don't let yourself be bullied into doing something scary that you don't really want to try. So what if someone thinks you're chicken? Stay true to what your own safety boundaries are.

doomed. This same technique can be used to calm yourself on an airplane flight that feels a bit too bumpy. Look at the flight attendants. If they seem okay with what is happening, it is probably not a dangerous situation.

How to Know If You Should Pack an Umbrella

Are you on the go all the time? We're guessing you are on the way out the door right now for a nice Sunday afternoon bike ride. Did you have time to check the weather forecast? Hmm, no. What about a weather Web site? And wade through tons of numbers, maps, and allergy medicine ads just to find out what the temperature is right now, let alone in a few hours? What's a girl to do? Actually, Jennifer found a guy who just happens to be a closet meteorologist. He loves cloud charts, and anytime there's a tornado somewhere, he's revved up. And that weather satellite map is one click away on his computer. He loves weather, and loves to be the bearer of bad news when a storm is lurking on the horizon.

Here are some secrets he shared with her that might help you become your own weather girl. Now, keep in mind, these don't apply equally everywhere—the United States has a whole lot of different "climate zones." But there are some basic rules:

- First, the prevailing winds through most of the United States (except Hawaii) are west to east. So if the wind is coming from some other direction—notably the south or southeast—guess what? That means a "low-pressure system" lurks to the west. And what does that mean? "It's going to rain soon," Peter says. But if the wind is from the west or southwest, that usually means fair weather and warmer. If it's from the northwest, especially in winter (except on the West Coast), it means cooler weather.

- And about those clouds; no clouds or small puffy white "cotton ball" cumulus clouds means stable air and good weather, especially if the humidity is low. Clouds with gray bottoms or multiple layers of clouds mean bad stuff is in store.

Those funny sailors' poems are right: red sky at night, everything's all right, but red sky in morning, sailor's warning. Extra-high levels of moisture bring the red color . . . and the rain at the end of the day.

Now, these tips work if you stick your head out the door. If you have a little more time and a computer, check out the NOAA Geostationary Orbiting Satellite Server Web site (it's easier than it sounds). Go to www.goes.noaa.gov, find your region and the infrared ("IR") image, and bookmark it. You'll see patterns of rain clouds and storm systems moving toward you. Then you'll know about bad stuff before anyone else does.

How to Pitch a Tent

Maslow's Hierarchy of Needs clearly states shelter as a necessary component of maintaining life—so Justin Clarence taught Lynne. An avid white-water rafter and camper, Justin spent more time outdoors than inside. The open space nurtured his soul, as he put it. Lynne doesn't know where he is right now—probably guiding people down a river in South America during the winter and down the Colorado River in the summer. He taught Lynne a useful tool in case the need for shelter ever arises . . . or if she goes camping. In this case, Lynne didn't ask to learn; Justin insisted she learn. He was her mountain man, and she can't go to Tahoe these days without a wistful sigh.

Here's what you should bring for pitching a tent:

- Tent
- Flashlight
- Tarp
- Broom
- A few extra sets of hands

Read the directions that come with the tent. No one taught us this (they wouldn't be caught dead reading the damn directions; of course they know how to put it up), but it really is mission-critical in our book. And this is our book, damn it. Read, study the diagram, and never throw it away. You might also want to have a practice run in the backyard before the trip if you think you need it. It helps to become familiar with the tent size and shape and to find out if any tent poles are missing.

Before you leave, check the weather forecast. If there's a good chance of rain or strong winds, bring the necessary extras that you would need, including extra stakes, rope, and tarps. If, unfortunately, you do encounter rain, pitching the tent under trees will help provide coverage. If the forecasts predict strong storms and possibly lightning, just don't camp. Why put yourself in a miserable and potentially dangerous position.

GETTING PREPARED

Make sure that you pitch the tent before sundown. Once night falls, even Grizzly Adams couldn't help you pitch that thing. And as much as you might want to imbibe, please pass around the booze *after* you pitch the tent. Otherwise you might end up naked in another family's fire pit a few sites over.

PICKING THE SPOT

When you arrive at your designated campsite, make sure to find the perfect spot. By "perfect," we mean with a minimal amount of rocks and other debris on the surface. If you scored a site on the coast, do anything you can to get the view. "My doctor said that it soothes my PMS if I watch the sunrise over the ocean." Nobody second-guesses PMS.

CLEANING THE AREA

With the broom we told you to pack, sweep the area clean of anything that might poke through the bottom of the tent. If you forgot a broom, no worries! A simple foot sweep would suffice. Or you can be a real outdoorswoman and find a fallen pine branch to use as a natural broom.

PITCHING THE TENT

Once the tent area is clean, lay the tarp down. Now you're ready to start pitching your tent:

1. Take everything out of the tent bag. You should have the following: a tent, a top cover, stakes, and poles connected with rope. Your bag might even have a picture of what the pitched tent looks like.

2. Find the tent and lay it flat on the tarp, considering where you want the opening to be. If your PMS excuse worked, the opening will face a gorgeous coastline.

3. If you're working with an average-size tent, the pack will have three sets of small poles. Take a group of small poles and start connecting them. Each one should fit into the other until you have three slightly wobbly poles.

. Stick one long pole through one of the openings on the edge

4. Stick one long pole through one of the openings on the edge of the tent. As you start pushing it across, there will usually be small hooks that clip onto the pole, and toward the middle of the tent will be sleeves. Stick the pole all the way across until it is correctly fitted on the other side.

5. Repeat that same process with the two other poles, making sure that the tent is still laying flat on the ground.

6. This is where you might want to call over some friends to get this baby standing. There should be small metal hooks at the edges of the tent where the poles come out. Stick the hooks into the end sides of the poles, making sure to do this one pole at a time. The poles should start forming half-circles in the air.

7. Now that the tent is up, find those stakes to keep the tent in place. After all, nobody likes to come back from a hike and find his or her tent rolling down the trail into the nearest bonfire.

8. Your tent should have something like loops around the edges for the stakes to go. Using a hammer or something similar, pound the stakes into the ground.

If this seems too tricky for your uptown-girl persona, there is such a thing as a self-pitching tent. You can pick one up at any sporting goods or camping store.

How to Light Up the Sky

When Lynne's friend Stev Zachary shops for fireworks, he's just like a kid in a candy store. Once, just days away from the Fourth of July in Cocoa, Florida, Lynne promised Stev that he could buy whatever fireworks he wanted. And that he could set them off on the dock by another friend's house on the Indian River. She didn't realize that this seemingly mellow, professional soccer player and sensitive sculptor possessed a side that she had never seen. She also learned a great deal about how to safely let off *real* fireworks—and what not to do as well.

Fireworks are not legal in all states or countries. Thankfully, many states, including Florida, sell fireworks year-round, including the real mortars that shoot two hundred feet into the air. Check with your home state to see whether you can host a barbecue and light up the night skies with awesome firepower any night of the week.

Did you know that when you buy professional-grade fireworks, you'll most likely sign a form stating that you will use them legally? It's a binding contract. Your name and address will be checked against identification and the fireworks traced back to you in the event of an "episode." By all means, rock and roll with the mortars—but do it within state and federal guidelines.

What is it about fire, fuses, and matches that intrigue men so much? From the time they're little, it's all about playing cowboys around the campfire and blowing up toy cars. Any action-adventure movie proves the point that men love explosions. But Lynne loves a great thriller like *Die Hard* and *The Transporter*, too. Why are women relegated to making the flag cake on the Fourth of July instead of setting off the fireworks? Lynne never had more fun in her entire life—including a trip to Europe—than the nights she and Stev blew up her best friend's front yard (and set a bottle rocket off inside the house, but we don't like to talk about that! It was an accident!). The adrenaline rush was out of this world. The key to this kind of fun, however, is ultimately knowing and using safety precautions. It quickly becomes no fun when someone loses a hand or an eye. For all you girls out there willing to take control of the fireworks festivities, here's the how-to.

PICK YOUR FIREPOWER

Before you ignite a single fuse, you must check your local and state rules regarding the use of fireworks. In California, for example, you'll never find *legal* fireworks with a bang and a light show unless you go to a controlled venue and sit with hundreds of other spectators. If you want the "light fantastic" closer to your home, you'll need to find the biggest badass fireworks available to you (and we'll tell you shortly how to make them appear even bigger and better). Some areas only have seasonal outlets that sell fireworks for a few weeks. Other areas have year-round stores that carry all your pyrotechnical desires. If you're not in the know, ask a salesperson. Some good "guylike" choices, however, that'll impress the hell out of any suitor are:

Anything that you can throw like a grenade or a rocket

Anything that you can use interactively

Any kind of propulsion device

Basically, ahem, bigger is better—big rocket, big torpedoes

PUT YOUR KNOWLEDGE TO WORK

Fireworks can break the bank. Don't obsess and let Roman candles rule your wallet. Shop wisely. Most fireworks establishments have two-for-one sales and lower prices closer to holidays. If you must play with pyrotechnics in March, prepare to spend some cash. Otherwise, channel your urge to light up the night sky until July, when prices plummet and sales abound.

PICK A SPOT

Plan where the fireworks display will occur. Look for places without foliage or fire hazards. Open spaces with concrete or dirt—good. The forest or jungle? Not good. Docks are always a good choice, and the reflection of the light bursting over the water is downright romantic. Do not, under any circumstances, set off fireworks from a boat. Choose someplace away from crowds, too. You'll have more fun if it's just you and a few friends anyway.

LIGHT UP THE NIGHT SKIES GUY STYLE

Plenty of legal fireworks are actually held and lit. The person who lights the fuses holds up the firework and shoots it into the sky. With a Roman candle, for example, bursts of light soar at intervals into the darkness, mimicking a lightning storm or a shooting star. Men often don't just hold the candle up and let it rip. Instead, they use the candle for imaginative play, where different stances flow with each burst and they become characters from their favorite action movies. First a ninja holds the firework, complete with "martial arts" speak. Next, "We got a bogey coming in to the left, Maverick," and suddenly everyone's in the movie *Top Gun*. Then Luke Skywalker emerges, protecting humanity with the good side of the Force. Of course, the duel begins as someone must play the role of the Sith Lord. *Star Wars* usually ends with pyrotechnic guitar wars. You get the idea. Instead of merely lighting the fuse, you, too, can enact an adventure.

In Stev's words, "You look at it like a really extravagant rave. Instead of the little glow sticks, you got the power."

Follow directions. Don't do anything ridiculous like load all twelve rockets in one canister and set it off on the concrete patio a few feet from guests! Don't shoot the fireworks directly at another person. Don't wait around after lighting the fuse, and always have a hose and a bucket to douse the used mortar, bottle rocket, or fire-cracker. By all means, play—just do it safely.

The best Stev gave Lynn? Light, let go, and run! Never grasp a firework that isn't meant to be held. A Roman candle, for example, is meant to be held. Most other fireworks are meant to be lit while on the ground, and your hands shouldn't touch them at all.

How to Draft a Fantasy Football Team

So your boyfriend says he wants you to play a much bigger role in his fantasy life. Cool! Then he asks for $20 and tells you to put on a football helmet. Should you worry? Probably not. Chances are he's just invited you to participate in his fantasy football league. We have both had to sit around listening to animated conversations about some fantasy football team or another. Once we finally got a handle on who was fantasizing about whom, it was much easier to put up with the endless (did we say endless?) discussions on the topic.

Here's the deal in a nutshell. In a fantasy football league you create a "team" by drafting (selecting) individual players from real NFL teams. The league is made up of eight to twelve other teams put together by friends and coworkers, all drafting from the same pool of players. Each week, you "play" against another team in the league. If the players on your team do better (statistically speaking) than the players on the other team, you win that game. At the end of the year, the team with the best win/loss record wins the season championship (and may be on the hook for hosting the postseason party!).

Fantasy football is a fun way to socialize through what might otherwise be a tediously long football season, but you'll need to do some homework before draft day and during the year to keep from ending up at the bottom of the standings. Here are some tips to get you started on the right foot:

- Drafting is the most important part of your game, since these are the guys you'll be stuck with for most of the year. You'll want to look at your league's previous year's results, or if it's a new league, go to one of the popular fantasy football league magazines like *Street & Smith's* to see how well players did last year.

- In most leagues you'll want to concentrate your early draft picks on running backs. These are the guys who'll be getting you most of your points, and good consistent scoring backs are the most valuable commodity in any league. Total yards are important, but a one-yard touchdown dive counts as much as a sixty-yard run. Look for guys who get the ball around the goal line.

- Avoid the temptation to take a famous quarterback (QB) or receiver/wide receiver (WR) too early; the difference between the best running back (RB) and an average running back is

Terms you need to know:

RB: Running back, also known as a halfback—the guy the quarterback gives the ball to once play begins.

QB: Quarterback—the guy who receives the ball after the snap from the center and tries to throw it or hand it off to a team member.

WR: Wide receiver—another one of the guys who goes out for a pass from the quarterback.

TE: Tight end—the guy who blocks sometimes and other times goes for a receiving route.

much greater than the difference between the best quarter-back and the tenth-best quarterback. Your first six rounds should go something like RB-RB-RB/QB-WR/RB-WR/QB-RB/QB, with at least three of those being RBs. Save the second half of the draft for your backups and a couple of place kickers.

- Most leagues allow you to "carry" as many as twenty players on your roster, which gives you a lot of flexibility and back-ups in case one of your starters gets injured. Each week you'll activate around ten players from your roster, including one quarterback, two or three running backs, two or three receivers, including a receiver, a tight end, a place kicker, and a team defense.

Your activation choices during the season will end up driving you crazy, so prepare yourself. Every week you'll have somebody on your starting team who plays badly and someone on your backups who has a huge day. Just get used to it and play the averages each week. You don't want to make wholesale changes to your basic starting lineup (unless you really blew your draft!), but if you have a good backup WR who's playing against a team that has a partic-ularly bad pass defense, it might be a good week to take a chance on him.

Don't be too concerned with winning; just have fun. Remem-ber, half the league loses every week. When you win, though, you have a seven-day pass to talk smack, so take advantage.

How to Play Beer Pong

There are men who can teach you about cognac and literature, and then there are men who can teach you how to play beer pong. How do we know this? We prefer not to say. But here's how to play:

Step 1: Get Everything You Need

- At least six beers, whatever kind you prefer.

- Enough water to fill two cups; it doesn't matter what kind.

- At least fourteen plastic cups (you can use regular cups, but who really wants to do dishes?).

- A Ping-Pong table (hence the name beer *pong*).

- Two Ping-Pong balls.

- A friend or more to play (drinking alone is not a good habit).

Step 2: Set Up the Game

- Place six cups at each end of the Ping-Pong table, in a triangular formation like pool balls. Have the row of three closest to your end of the table and make sure that each cup is touching the adjacent cup.

- Open your beers and poor approximately half a can or bottle into four of the cups.

- Fill the two remaining cups with water. (Balls are most likely going to hit the ground, and let's face it, you probably don't clean your Ping-Pong table every day, so these cups are used to clean off the balls between throwing.)

- Have each player take his or her place at opposite ends of the table.

Step 3: The Rules

- To start off, the winner shoots first. If it's the first game, the players stare at their opponent's eyes and on the count of three throw a ball. The first player to sink a cup gets to go first. If both players make it, they keep shooting until only one player makes it.

- Each player gets to throw two balls per turn. If a player makes both her shots, she gets the balls back and receives an extra turn.

- The player has the choice of either throwing or bouncing the ball into a cup. Standard rules prohibit having your elbow over the edge of the table, but you can determine with your opponent before the game if you want to permit leaning over.

- When a player successfully gets a ball into an opponent's cup, it is considered "sunk," and the opponent must drink its contents.

- Toward the end of the game, when a player has come down to her last cup and the opponent sinks it, the losing player earns what's called "rebuttal": a chance to stay in the game. The losing player gets another turn to try and sink the opponent's remaining cups. Just as with a regular turn, if she sinks two in a row, she gets another turn. If the rebuttal is successful, the game goes into overtime.

- In overtime three cups are set up in a triangle. The player who was winning gets the first turn, and another standard game is played.

Now that you know the rules, it's time to lock eyes with your opponent and get those Ping-Pong balls flying. Good luck and always remember to drink responsibly.

How to Play Ultimate Frisbee

Why not spend your afternoons watching tanned and toned men running around on a field? Jennifer enjoys it tremendously; she watches her husband, Peter, play a game called Ultimate Frisbee. Invented in the 1960s on a college campus, Ultimate Frisbee is a groovy underground and somewhat disorganized sport that has grown popular on college campuses, in high-tech businesses, and with venture capitalists in California's Silicon Valley. Her husband learned to play at Hewlett-Packard, and it took Jennifer the longest time to figure out what those sweaty guys were actually doing as they ran up and down the field after a Frisbee. Although many nonplayers assume that it is somehow related to the laid-back game of Frisbee golf, it is nothing like it. Instead, Ultimate is a thorough mind-body exercise, played by smart people, combining speed, endurance, strength, and a modest amount of motor coordination into a safe, noncontact game that's actually fun to play. And it costs practically nothing. So in case you also have to spend time sitting in the grass watching some guys run back and forth, here is what they are doing:

Ultimate got its start in New Jersey as the "ultimate sports experience" sometime in the late 1960s. It's a team sport (there are between three and seven players on a team) that is played on a field similar to a football field with end zones and sidelines.

The disc (a 175-gram Frisbee, kind of big but not hard to handle) is moved down the field by throwing it to other members of your team. You can't run with the disc. Team members throw, catch, throw, catch until successfully throwing it to someone on their team in the end zone. That's a score.

Play doesn't stop until someone scores. If the disc is dropped, intercepted, or otherwise not caught in bounds, it's a turnover and play starts immediately going the other direction—again, until a score. Once someone picks up the disc, he has a ten count to throw it, measured off by a marker, or defender, guarding them.

The exercise comes from constant motion trying to get open for a throw on offense or playing defense, trying to shut down the other team's throws. It's man-on-man (well, person-on-person) defense across the whole field; there are no "positions" as such.

And here's what's so great—it's fun. Ultimate combines the best of hockey, basketball, and soccer into a safe sport requiring modest skill. And it's a good place to show your creativity, by curving throws or throwing an over-the-top hammer. You'll also learn a forehand flick, sort of a field version of a baseball infielder's throw to first base.

It's a great coed game, and women's and coed Ultimate is played at a collegiate and club level throughout the world. Ultimate is played by cool people, usually those looking for an alternative to typical "ball" sports, jocks, nitpicky rules, and referees. There are no officials, and it's pretty social, with lots of talk on the field.

If you want to get out and play with the guys you may have to trim your fingernails a little—the game's a bit hard on them. And you'll have to be patient as you gain the "wheels" (endurance) and perfect some of the basic throws. You'll have to buy a pair of cleated shoes (soccer shoes will work). Other than shorts and a T-shirt, little else is needed to get started, except a group to play with. You may have to search a little for a group or a club playing in your area, but the Internet is great for that. Also check out the Ultimate Players Association Web site (www.upa.org) to learn more about the game and where to play in your area. You'll get all the exercise you need, for all parts of your body, with no sore knees or quads. It's exhilarating and fun! Even Jennifer gets up off the blanket she puts at the edge of the field to watch and joins in once in a while.

How to Hike to the Top of a Big Mountain

What kind of a nut would look at a big, tall mountain and think, "Hmm . . . wonder what the view is from up there?" Lots of guys Jennifer dated, that's who. Including the one she married, Peter, who finally nagged her into one of America's toughest hikes: Yosemite's Half Dome. Okay, so the view was pretty nice from up there, but there is a real art and skill to getting there. And you can't just decide one day to tackle a long upward climb. Jennifer took many notes in the weeks she prepared for this seventeen-mile hike up a nine-thousand-foot mountain (it helped distract her from the task at hand).

Here are a few important things to know before you join your friends on a hike:

- **Don't wear new boots or old running shoes.** Your happiness and success throughout the day will depend almost entirely on whether your feet feel good, so take care beforehand to make sure that they will. Go out and buy a pair of actual hiking boots, and then wear them everywhere, all day long, for at least two weeks. Do not buy them the day before. Do not buy them the week before and then leave them in the box until you get up that morning to hike. No, we really do want you to wear them for long stretches at a time to break them in and get used to them. And even better if you can take small hikes or fast walks in them a few times before the big event.

- **Don't bring along any equipment you haven't already tried.** Not just the boots (see above) but also hiking poles, camelbacks, binoculars, digital cameras, whatever. The dusty trail up a mountain is not the place to learn how to use something new. Before climbing Half Dome, Jennifer even practiced unzipping her hiking pants to turn them into shorts and taking the pant legs off over her boots. Of course she looked silly doing this on a nature trail near her house, but hey, she was able to do it without falling over when she needed to later on.

- **Recognize your body's need for fuel.** Sure, you are going to buy one of those cool camelback thingies that you can fill with three liters of water and sip when you need it. Please do; they are great. But also make sure that you carry a few treats like almonds, raisins, GORP, and even hard candy to suck on for a quick sugar boost. Bring along a peanut butter and jelly sandwich for lunch, but don't be surprised if you don't feel that hungry for a big meal with the adrenaline of the adventure running through you. Later, after the hike is behind you, you will be ravenous, but on the trail you might not be and might have to remember to keep eating a bit now and then anyway.

- **Train on stadium stairs.** Even long and strenuous hikes won't really get your body ready for an uphill climb unless they, too, are headed uphill. The best way to get your body ready to climb is to climb. And since few of us live in the mountains, instead head to a school with a large stadium and start to climb up and down the stands. You could also train by climbing the stairs in tall office buildings, and more than one serious mountaineer has gotten ready for Mount Everest in an office park with plentiful stairs and steps.

- **Be adventurous, but don't take risks.** Don't let someone goad you into doing something your body isn't ready for or your spirit isn't up for. And by all means don't let anyone make you do something that doesn't feel safe.

How to Play Poker

Lynne's friend Rhonda is currently dating a poker dealer. Before he started dealing, he played most every Friday night. When you fall for a card dealer, you learn that you either stay home most weekends or play poker. Consequently, she played poker. Rhonda learned so well from her male friends and boyfriend that she's swiftly working her way up to the World Poker Tour and continues to win in money games all over the country. Poker seems to be a sport dominated by men, so learn how to hedge your bets and you might find a mate for life who loves the way you play!

While whole books are devoted to poker, you don't need them. You just need brains and a few basics. And while many different poker games exist, all possess the same conclusion: the best five-card hand wins.

One of the most popular games is No Limit Texas Hold 'Em. Before even beginning to play, you need to memorize and learn the rankings of hands from highest to lowest. It's best to learn these hands and play against a few friends to get comfortable with your stride, poker face, and confidence.

PUT YOUR KNOWLEDGE TO WORK

Ever wonder why you see the guys on television in the big poker tournaments showing no emotion—even wearing sunglasses to hide their eyes? They don't want anyone to sense or see whether they're excited about a big hand or bluffing. Great bluffers can win the pot even if they have a bad hand. If you push everyone out because they're afraid you have a royal flush when all you really have is a nonsuited two and seven, you win. But adept players know the "tells," or quirks, that people they play with consistently "show." Rhonda's boyfriend swears he now knows that she does something with her eyebrows when she's bluffing and twitches her eyes when she's not. Pay attention to the hands people play and their manners. And become aware of your body language. Lynne knows a player who continually looks at her cards with both good and bad hands, as if she's forgotten what she's holding. This tactic makes it impossible for anyone to read the gal. When you play, find your own way to bluff.

The Basics

- Know the suits: clubs, hearts, diamonds, and spades.
- The highest hand is a **Royal Flush**: ace, king, queen, jack, ten, all of the same suit. In the rare case when two or more players hold all same suit cards, the suits rank highest to lowest, like this: spades, clubs, diamonds, hearts.
- The next best hand is the **Straight Flush**: five cards in sequence with the same suit. Even if you're holding two, three, four, five, six of clubs, you can win over the next-best hand.
- What is next? **Four of a Kind**: four cards of the same number or rank (by rank, we mean ace, king, queen, and jack), and one other card.
- **Full House** comes next: three cards of the same number or rank (called a triple) and two of the same number or rank (called a pair).
- The next winner under a Full House is the **Flush**: five cards of the same suit in no particular order. You might be holding king, seven, five, three, two, and if they're all in diamonds, you might be the winner.
- Next up, the **Straight**: five cards, any suit, in sequence. Higher straights (such as queen, jack, ten, nine, eight) beat lower straights (such as six, five, four, three, two).
- **Three of a Kind** comes next: three cards of the same rank or number. For example, three queens, three sevens, three twos. If no one has a better hand, you win—even with the three twos (better known as deuces).
- **Two Pair** comes next: two cards of the same number or rank and another two cards with the same number or rank. A pair of queens and a pair of sevens is an example of this hand.
- Next is a **Pair**: two cards of the same number or rank.

- Last is **High Card**: if no one has any of the previous hands, the person with the highest card wins.

How to Play No Limit Texas Hold 'Em

- You receive two cards from the dealer that no one sees but you, then the betting begins. You either bet the minimum blind (the lowest bet) or raise it, depending upon how strongly you feel about your hand. Remember, you have no idea what the dealer will lay down or what the other players are holding.

- Once each player bets, the dealer lays down the flop, consisting of three cards faceup. These are the community cards and can be used by everyone to help his or her original hand. More betting around the table ensues.

- Now, here's where it gets crazy. When it's your turn to bet, you have four options. (1) You can fold, which means that you give your two original cards back to the dealer and you're out of the hand. (2) You can check, which means that you are not putting any more money into the pot, but you're still in the hand. (3) You can call, which means that you will bet the same amount that the previous player bet. (4) Or finally, you can raise the previous player's bet in the hopes that others will fold. Others may also raise and re-raise in order to push out players with weak hands or to increase the pot.

> **Extra Credit**
>
> When a player checks, she doesn't put money into the pot—she bets nothing. In the beginning of the game, when players are trying to determine if they have a chance, they'll often check until the flop is dealt. Once the flop lands, you'll have a better idea if any of your cards can make a hand, and the real betting begins.

- The dealer then deals the fourth community card, also known as the "turn."

- Everyone bets, checks, calls, or folds. If you stay in, it's called "taking it to the river," to see the last faceup card by the dealer.

- Once the fifth and final community card, the "river," is dealt, the betting ensues. If two or more players are left in the game at this point, they must show their cards to determine who has the highest hand and rakes in the chips. This is known as the showdown.

- If everyone folds but one person, that person automatically wins the pot and doesn't have to show his or her hand. That way, no one knows if the winner was bluffing! Often the goal of Texas Hold 'Em is not to get to the showdown but to make people fold before the hand is over. The less information you provide other players—in the form of twitches, eye blinks, and so on—the more chances you have of keeping your bluffing "tells" a secret . . . and winning more!

Pocket rockets are two aces. Initially, one might think it's a great hand, and technically, it is the strongest possible pre-flop hand. But even so, the odds of winning with pocket rockets is only one in three, so don't bet the farm if you find yourself holding two of these babies. Your rockets might crash.

The best thing you can possibly do in learning how to play poker is to get together with a few people who know how to play and will patiently teach you during the informal game. Get help mastering the hands and your chances will improve greatly. From there, find locations with games where you tip the dealer $5 to $10 each game to play. These games earn you certificates toward the "buy in" to big-money tournaments. Basically, you need to prove yourself in smaller games. Earning a certain number of certificates will garner you a seat in a tournament. Remember, girls, men might seem to dominate the sport, but the big winner at the World Series of Poker Tournament in 2006, Annie Duke, was a young mother!

How to Throw a Punch

Lynne probably shouldn't be as proud as she is about it, but many a man has thrown a few punches over the years in defense of her honor. The boyfriend who taught her how he actually connected fist to chin did so when another man looked too closely at Lynne's upper torso in front of a restaurant. A girl needs to know how to throw a punch for more important reasons than stupid tiffs over looks. Girls should learn it as a self-defense measure.

Remember, in a brawl, there are no rules. If you enter it, commit to it.

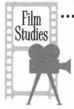

Film Studies

Why not learn more fighting technique from Brad Pitt in *Fight Club*? Even if you aren't that interested in perfecting your punch, you can spend the time watching Brad perfect his. There are worse ways to spend an evening.

The Basics

1. Don't begin with your body standing square in front of your opponent. Take a "Tae Bo" stance—sideways to your opponent, one foot slightly in front of the other.

2. Don't draw back with your punching arm. Keep both arms in close to your chest or more toward your face so you can block a punch if it comes at you first. Keep those arms close in to your frame.

3. Here's where it gets good. If you are right-handed, your left foot will be closer to your opponent. Step forward with the

left foot and use the momentum of your body, not your arm, to propel your right fist into the punch. If you are left-handed, do just the opposite.

 Never loop your arm back for a hook. It leaves you less defended and only relying on your arm strength. Throwing a punch has more effect when you use the momentum of your body.

4. Snap the punch quickly—jab it.

5. When your fist extends, it should be in a palm-down position, with your thumb on the outside.

6. Punch anywhere your opponent is undefended and vulnerable. If his hands are down and away from his face, slam the nose, jaw, ear, anything on the face. If his body is undefended, hit hard in the stomach area.

7. If your opponent isn't able to counter, keep moving forward; do not backpedal, and continue to attack until you feel safe enough to leave.

PUT YOUR KNOWLEDGE TO WORK

Although throwing the first punch may make you legally liable for assault, every man Lynne has ever spoken with regarding brawls says, "Be the aggressor if you know someone is in your face and planning on hurting you. Get at them when they're off guard to protect yourself." One guy even likened it to the fight-or-flight response. He said, "If you fly, chances are you'll get tackled and the last thing you want is to be on the ground where you can really get hurt." We hope you'll never need to throw a punch. And we assume no liability if you ever do decide to throw one.

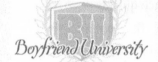

Boyfriend University

YOU'VE GRADUATED!

So many men, so little time to learn everything! At least now you've graduated from Boyfriend University with a breadth of knowledge. Whether you need to quickly make a killer spaghetti or know when to call a man, we've tried to help you on your relationship journey. Men are amazing creatures. We love them. We hope that in some way, this book has helped you to appreciate the guys in your life—and appreciate how beautiful, powerful, and interesting you are, too.

And please do visit our Web site, www.boyfriend university.com. We want to hear what your boyfriend taught you!

Index

Index

Index

Index

Index

Printed in the USA
CPSIA information can be obtained
at www.ICGtesting.com
LVHW091513080824
787695LV00001B/88

9 780470 177037